15-150 Secret to Simple Dieting

15-150 Secret to Simple Dieting

Dr. Steven Rosenberg and Bobbie Freiberg

To order additional copies of this book, contact:
Xlibris Corporation
1-888-795-4274
www.Xlibris.com
Orders@Xlibris.com
73073

CONTENTS

ACKNOWLEDGMENTS

Photography By: Tetra Strategic Communications

Food Stylist: Chef Andreas Makris

Cover Design: Andrew Fiorentino

CHAPTER 1

INTRODUCTION

It's easy to gain weight in America. With all the fast-food and chain restaurants, not to mention a pizza place in every shopping center, eating fattening food is cheaper and more convenient than ever. Living as we do in a country where hamburgers are among the cheapest foods, everything comes with fries, and you can buy a sandwich that uses fried chicken in place of a bun, it's no surprise that being overweight is so prevalent.

That's not to say that our society isn't taking steps to correct this unhealthy situation. Lately, there has been a push to include calorie listings on restaurant menus. That helps; unfortunately, calories don't tell the whole story. If you go to the movies or a baseball game and the only choices are high-calorie foods, how does the calorie listing help? Fattening foods can be so tasty and are so easily available at all times of day that it's easy to ignore the calories when you're looking for a quick fix on your break from work or a meal at the ball game or something to feed a family of four on a budget.

Once you've gained the weight, it can be very difficult to lose. Many people try to diet and exercise, but even if you are very committed, it can be tough. First, you have to pick the right diet for you—not just to make you lose weight but also to keep you healthy. You may have to deal with giving up foods you love. You may have to get all your meals shipped to you in microwaveable containers and plastic bags, and that's just not very appetizing. We don't blame you if you don't want to eat chicken or ravioli or risotto that you got in the mail. Even if you successfully lose weight, you may not know how to maintain your weight loss, causing you to gain all that weight back.

All this can take a major toll on your mental and physical health. Our bodies were not meant to carry all the extra weight that so many of us are carrying, and it can make us feel horrible physically. Extra weight makes us more prone to joint and muscle pains, diabetes, heart disease, liver disease, breathing problems, strokes, and cancer—just to name a few. That's in the long term.

Right now, as you wake up overweight every day, it's stressful to feel like you can't do the things you were once able to when you were thinner. Dieting itself can be stressful and discouraging, particularly if you have trouble following the diet or it doesn't work for you, and that stress can actually bring you back to food, making you add extra pounds.

So it's understandable if you've come to think that there's no way you're ever going to lose weight and keep it off. Maybe you think you can't afford it; maybe you think your lifestyle doesn't support it; maybe you just like all the fat and the additives that make fast food taste good. No matter what the reason, Americans have become the most overweight people in the world.

Obesity is steadily overtaking smoking as the top health issue in our country, but even though we hear about it, we don't do much about it. Amid all the debate about government-run health care, it's easy to miss that the person with the greatest control over your health is you. You have the power to make yourself into the person you want to be—that power just needs to be harnessed and used.

But if you're holding this book, you've already found the way to lose those pounds and live a healthier lifestyle. We are going to show you that you *can* eat tasty healthy food without overspending, and it's easier than you might think.

In this book, you will find a diet that is absolutely, scientifically 100 percent guaranteed to work You're going to get help putting yourself in the right frame of mind to stick to the plan so you can achieve your weight goal. You are going to find out how you can have a healthy lifestyle while still being able to eat great foods. You are going to achieve all this with

Now, some of the hospital staffers already were in the practice of reading labels, but they weren't looking for the right things. Several of them had tried high-protein, low-carb diets, which do work but are not ideal for women. That kind of diet works well for men's weight loss, but women who try it typically lose weight and then gain it back once they start eating carbs again.

Cutting carbs from your diet almost entirely is unsustainable—you can do it for a while, but you can't avoid carbs forever—so it's not a long-term solution. Additionally, according to a recent study, those high-fat, low-carb diets can actually negatively affect the dieter's mood and are not more effective than low-fat, high-carb diets.[1] The 15/150 diet finds a happy medium by controlling both fat and carbs, but leaving enough carbs in your diet to keep you burning energy efficiently and, equally important, to keep you in a positive state of mind.

Diets that cut your caloric intake to very low levels can help you lose weight in the short term but also leave you feeling hungry and less energetic. The key is to find healthy foods that are low in fat and fairly low in carbohydrates while still eating enough productive calories, not empty calories from sugar—that you feel good about yourself and sustain your energy level.

So our goal was to create a situation where these hospital staffers could eat some carbohydrates but still limit their intake of carbs and fat in a way that would allow them to lose weight and feel good about themselves. You can do that with two simple numbers: 15 and 150. That is the crux of this diet. Through extensive research, I have determined that if you eat no more than 15 g of fat and no more than 150 g of carbohydrates per day, you are scientifically guaranteed to lose weight.

In my years as a science teacher, I'd worked with a calorimeter in my classes. A calorimeter is used to measure the heat generated by chemical processes. More specifically, I used a heat-loss calorimeter. A heat-loss calorimeter has a space inside it in which chemical reactions take place. The heat inside that space, or cell, is collected by a copper cup, which

---

[1]   "Long-term Effects of a Very Low-Carbohydrate Diet and a Low-Fat Diet on Mood and Cognitive Function." *Arch Intern Med.* 2009;169(20):1873-1880.

conducts it through a layer of silicone rubber, which works as a thermal resistor, conducting the heat to an outer copper cup, which is filled with constantly flowing water. This allows us to accurately measure, in a laboratory environment, how the substance within the calorimeter is burning, then observe how completely it has burned.

Using my knowledge of the calorimeter, I conducted a series of experiments to determine what burns best and most completely in the body. What I found was that lower-fat and lower-carb foods are actually anti-inflammatory foods, and they burn more completely in your body. If you can create a situation where your diet is composed of relatively low-carb and low-fat foods, your body will burn that food more efficiently. You may not even have realized that anti-inflammatory foods exist; they are like anti-inflammatory medications and are actively good for your body in ways besides weight loss.

Inflammation—including pain, redness, and swelling inside your body—can be caused or exacerbated by foods that are very high in fat, carbohydrates, and nitrates. Eating anti-inflammatory foods that are low in fat and carbohydrates can, in addition to reducing your weight, help reduce painful inflammation you're experiencing without medication.

With my calorimeter experiments, I was able to determine that the optimal levels for the best and cleanest anti-inflammatory burn are 15 g to 20 g of fat and 150 g to 200 g of carbohydrates on a daily basis. In order to lose weight, it's best to be on the low end of that; to maintain weight loss, we take the numbers up a notch, as we'll discuss in the section on maintenance. As long as you monitor your fat and carb intake and keep it down, you're going to do well.

In the case of the hospital staffers and the approximately one thousand people who have come to me over the past eight years, they have indeed done very well. Everyone has lost weight. Everyone has kept the weight off. That can be attributed to the best aspect of this diet: it's a lifestyle, and it's easy to stick to it because you're not going to feel like you're denying yourself. All you've got to do is stick to reading labels and stay within the 15 and 150 numbers.

Fortunately, nutrition labels are now easier to read, and more people are reading them than ever before. Because people are learning to read labels and are demanding better food, companies have learned to make healthier versions of the foods and drinks we've come to love. When the hospital staffers came to me, I devised for them a shopping list with lower-fat, lower-carb foods that they would enjoy and be able to eat while losing weight and not feeling deprived of food quality or quantity.

In this book, I'm going to expand on that with a little bit of help from a patient, who was so thrilled with her weight loss on the 15/150 diet, that she wrote the second half of this book. Together, we're going to teach you how to eat well so you can lose weight and keep it off. But more importantly, we're going to teach you a lifestyle that will make you feel better about yourself and everything around you. After all, there are a million diets. The challenge for dieters is finding one that works and sticking to it. That's just what we're going to help you do.

CHAPTER 3
SELF-LIMITING BELIEFS

"Diets make me feel deprived and hungry."

"Yeah, I can lose weight, but I'm only going to gain it back and then gain more."

"My parents are overweight, so it's in my genes."

"If it hasn't happened yet, it never will."

"If I get my hopes up too high, I'll only get hurt."

"People will make fun of me for being on a diet."

"I'm not good enough."

"Somebody or something will always stand in the way of my success."

Statements like these are called self-limiting beliefs because that is precisely what they do: these thoughts are capable of making us unwilling or unable to improve ourselves. Before we begin any lifestyle change, it's critical to rid ourselves of the self-limiting beliefs that can hold us back.

All of the thoughts above have been cited to me by my patients as reasons that they'll never lose weight, and they're only a small sampling of the reasons people think they won't be able to make a diet work. You might believe that looking better will change your personality for the worse, damage your relationships with your friends, or inspire new romantic relationships that will end in heartache. All these beliefs can make you afraid to let your hopes get too high for fear of disappointment. The fear of failure, after all, is a very powerful one; that's where pretty much all of our inhibitions come from. With our help, you're going to adopt a positive, can-do attitude. But there's no need to be afraid of failing to lose weight; what you should truly be afraid of is failing to try.

If you've got self-limiting beliefs, it's not your fault. It can be hard to find the right situation for weight loss, and you can have trouble achieving the results you want. You may have tried other diets before and lost weight but been unable to keep it off. You may have simply been unable to stick to a diet plan; everyone's got their own life to live, and overly specific diets can fall by the wayside.

But you should never hold yourself back, not with weight loss and not with anything you want to achieve in life. Life is too short for you to be your own worst enemy. Confront your negative beliefs, clear them from your mind, and replace them with positive thoughts. You are capable and worthy of achieving your goals, and there is no reason to be discouraged from believing that. If you believe in yourself, nothing will keep you from accomplishing what you set out to do.

Beyond the science, any diet can only be as good as the dieter. So even though this diet is extremely simple, like any other diet, it requires a commitment from the dieter to stick to it and to avoid fattening foods. Ensuring that you follow through with your diet is just as important to me as getting you on it in the first place.

Regardless of your position in life, there isn't any outside factor that is strong enough to overcome your willpower and your desire to lose weight and feel better about yourself. This book is intended to help you focus your willpower, bring it to bear, and apply it in a way that will increase the quality of your life. The 15/150 regimen is so easy to follow that you'll surprise yourself with how naturally you pick it up once you get those nasty self-limiting beliefs out of your way.

One great technique that will help you clear those negative, self-limiting beliefs is to complete a little homework that I give to my patients. Go get a poster board or foam board, lay it down on your desk or another flat surface, and find pictures of you or things or foods that you feel are important in order to move you forward and out of the rut of self-limiting beliefs. Put on a picture of yourself from back when you were at an ideal weight level. If you don't have one, find a picture of someone else with the body type you want to reach.

Add pictures of foods that you know are healthy that you can eat and enjoy. Add words or phrases that are important or inspirational to you—15/150 should be on there somewhere. The idea of low fat, low carbs, staying on the program—all the positive thoughts that you can put down—throw them on that board in the form of pictures, words, and phrases that are important and meaningful to you. Then put it somewhere very visible to you so that you see it throughout the day.

When you look at this collage, you are going to think about getting past those self-limiting beliefs, moving forward, and getting yourself out of that psychological rut of feeling that you are incapable of losing weight. This poster board represents where you're going and what you're going to achieve with the 15/150 diet and your new attitude.

The program written out in the next chapter is similar to the one I give to my patients on an individual basis and will help you get rid of those self-limiting beliefs. The program involves the use of a relaxation technique that with repetition, allows you to change habits and behaviors. The relaxation program will allow you to ingrain positive thought processes (PTPs) into your mind. Putting those positive thought processes in your head will allow you to really move forward and feel good about succeeding in what you want to do and what you want to accomplish.

Perhaps the most important positive thought process for you to keep in your mind is not to get discouraged no matter what happens. These are big changes you're making in your life, so even if you ease into them, it's very possible that something will happen—perhaps something stressful will come up, and you'll experience a moment of weakness—and you will break from the diet one day, eating something rife with fat and carbohydrates. So many dieters have stopped because they broke their diet one day. The stress of it can be very powerful; it can be very discouraging. Do not give up. Use the exercises in the following chapter to calm yourself. Stay positive. You may have stepped off the trail for a moment, but you can get right back on it.

You have the power.

CHAPTER 4

DR. ROSENBERG'S SNOOZE TO LOSE

This is a slightly modified version of a program that I do for my patients. Ordinarily, I record this on a CD during a session and send the CD home with my patient, but because we were unable to include a CD with this version of the book, we have included this relaxation session in text form for you to practice at home.

Sit or lie down somewhere comfortable and have someone read this to you. You can also read it to yourself, but it won't work nearly as well. It will be most effective if someone (preferably someone with a calming voice) reads this to you so that you can really just let it take hold. This is about harnessing the powers of your own mind to enable you to control your body, and as such, it's better if you can keep your mind clear of the distraction of reading.

Try to practice this every day. If you don't have someone who can read this to you every day, then record someone, even yourself, reading it and play it back for yourself. If you would prefer, a pre-recorded version of my CD will be available from our website. This will help you overcome stress and stick to your diet.

To help you gain control over your eating habits and your eating desires, I would like you to get into a very comfortable and relaxed position. Stare directly at the object in front of you. Keep your eyes wide open, and as you stare, as you gaze, as you focus, and as you concentrate, you will begin to feel the air circulating around the room, hitting your open eyes. Your eyes will become dry and tired. It's only natural that when you stare at an object the way you're staring now, your eyes will want to close more and more. Your eyes are beginning to burn and tear—that's only natural. Your eyes are becoming heavy, burning, stinging, and wanting to close more and more.

Now I'm going to count from five backward to one, and as each number becomes smaller, your eyes will want to close more and more, and finally on the count of one, I would like you to just close your eyes and relax them.

Five, the eyes are burning; four, wanting to close more and more, getting very, very heavy; three, getting very fatigued; two, getting ready to close now. And on the count of one, just close your eyes. Allow the eyes to remain closed until I ask you to open them later.

This is now your time, your private time, your time to use the powers of your own mind to help you to do well. And I would like you to relax your entire body and to clear your mind. To help you do that, I would like you to repeat silently, mentally, to yourself the following phrases of relaxation.

My mind is quite quiet. My mind is clear. I feel that relief of closing my eyes spread into my forehead. I am able to wipe away all of those lines and creases in my forehead, and that relief is moving into my scalp then into the back of my neck and my shoulders. My arms are very, very heavy. My hands are relaxed and loose. And I am able to feel that relief of closing my eyes move downward into my cheeks and my chin. My chest muscles are so very, very heavy. My abdomen is relaxed and loose. All of the large and small muscles in my back are so relaxed. My hips, my thighs, and even my knees are relaxed. My calf muscles are so very, very heavy. The bottoms of my feet and even my toes are relaxed.

And I begin to drift away—I float away. I dream. I sleep. I let go. I clear my mind. It is my subconscious mind that I want to reach, and I am able to do that by counting backward from twenty down to zero. Every number that I count backward will take my body deeper and deeper, and when I reach the count of zero, I will become deeply relaxed, deeply subconscious. I will be deep asleep.

Twenty, I go deeper and deeper; nineteen, deeper still. Eighteen, every breath takes my body deeper and deeper. Seventeen, I am relaxing more and more. I feel wonderful. Sixteen, my mind is clear; fifteen, deeply meditating; fourteen, thoroughly relaxed; thirteen, deeper. Twelve, every breath hits my body deeper and deeper. Eleven, ten, I'm deeply relaxed; nine, eight, seven, going deeper and deeper; six, five, becoming deep asleep; four, three, two, going down deeper and deeper; one, even deeper. Zero. Deep asleep. Deeply relaxed. Deeply subconscious.

It is my subconscious mind that is working for me to help me, and I realize now that I want to lose weight and I have the ability to do this. I have the ability to do anything that I really want to do. I know that I should be eating healthfully and I am able to do that by reading the labels of every food that I purchase. I will eat as little fat as I possibly can. In fact, I will eat no more than fifteen grams of fat total for the entire day. That means I will stay away from those high-fat foods. I will stay away from butter and margarine, each of which is eleven grams of fat per tablespoon. I will stay away from oil, real mayonnaise, real salad dressings, and peanut butter, each of which is seven to eleven grams of fat per tablespoon.

I will stay away from all eggs. The yolk is five grams of fat by itself. There is no fat in the white. I will stay away from red meat. One ounce of red meat can have nine grams of fat. I will stay away from cheeses. One slice, one ounce, of cheese can be up to thirteen grams of fat. And I will eat no more than fifteen grams of fat for the entire day.

I will limit my carbohydrate intake to no more than 150 g total for the entire day. That means I will stay away from those things that are high in carbohydrates. That means I will stay away from soda and energy drinks. One serving of a nondiet energy drink or soda has 25 to 35 g of carbohydrates. I will stay away from white bread, which has 15 g of carbs in a slice. I will control my intake of corn and potatoes, which are very high in carbs. And I will eat no more than 150 g of carbohydrates for the entire day.

And I can do it. I have the ability to do it. I am worth it. I am worth that effort. I want to be thinner and trimmer. Food is secondary to me. Food is no longer that treat, nor is it that reward that it once was. I would much rather wear clothes of a smaller size and have them fit. I would much rather look in the mirror and like what is looking back at me.

Thinner, trimmer, and healthier—that is my object. And I am able to do it; I am so motivated to do that. I am ready to lose weight. And I am so proud of myself. I am proud to be me and proud to have this newfound discipline that I am able to put down those foods that I know I should not eat. I am able to put them down and not touch them. I know I will stay away from the junk foods, the excess carbs, and the sweets. I will stay away from the white-flour starches. I know that I can do this. I know that the way to lose weight is to eat lower fat, lower carbs, higher protein, and less white flour. I can do this. I have that newfound discipline within me, within my own mind and my body, and within my own heart. I know that I am able to do this. I am proud to be me, proud to be that special person, and proud to have that newfound discipline to really eat properly.

And I will drink the fluids that will allow me to really do well. Fluids are important to my general health and my well-being. I will drink as much fluid as possible. And I will drink one full glass of water before each and every meal.

And I will be more active. I can be more active, even if it is only taking stairs instead of elevators and escalators or parking my car farther from my destination so I have to walk more. I can be more active. I love being active. I love losing weight. And I can see in my mind that thinner, trimmer image of me. I see in my mind that thinner, trimmer image, and I love it. "Thin" is my key word to happiness.

I am in control. I am number one. I am that positive and very motivated person. I feel great about myself. I am so proud of me, proud to be me, and proud to be in control of my eating habits completely. I am that special person, special thanks to the fact that I have found that new discipline in me and that newfound motivation to really do well. I can do well. I am doing well. I am adhering to a very healthy eating habit. I can do it all. I am exercising to the best of my ability. I am drinking water. I am hydrating my body. Hydrating my body is so healthy for me.

And I see that image of me in my mind and I love it. Thinner, trimmer—that image is me. And every time that I work with this program, I will go deeper and deeper, and all of these ideas will become paramount to my mind. Every time that I work with this programming, these ideas will make an indelible imprint into my subconscious level, and I will do these things, and I will feel great. I will be healthy, vibrant, and positive. I am proud of myself—proud to be me.

And so I am going to count from one forward to five, and when I reach the count of five, I will ask you to just open your eyes and feel wonderful.

On the count of one, I feel the energy building now; two, coming up more and more, feeling great; three, positive and motivated to lose weight; four, coming up more and more, feeling wonderful, motivated, and strong. And on the count of five, just open the eyes and feel positive in every way, proud to be you—proud to be that special person and to be in control of your eating habits completely.

CHAPTER 5

GETTING INTO THE RIGHT
STATE OF MIND

We're going to keep this easy. If you've bought this book, you're already stressed out about your weight, about any previous dieting failures, or maybe about life in general. There's no need to stress you out more with a difficult diet or complicated lifestyle changes. After all, you might be overeating or unwilling to exercise because of all the stress in your life. So the first step toward freeing you from the discomfort and the unhealthiness of being overweight, even before we get into dieting, is to reduce your stress.

What stresses you out? Is it your job, your marriage, your children, your parents, or your financial situation? Even fun things can stress us out—packing and preparing for vacations, getting the family together for special occasions, and so on.

These stress-inducing factors are called stressors. No one will ever be able to rid themselves of all stressors, but that's okay because they're not all bad. Some people work better under stress, and some stress in general is good to create motivation and energy in us. Small amounts of stress can help improve our memories as well as help us work faster and better. When our stress becomes too powerful, however, we have to take steps to reduce it. You're going to learn in this chapter how to reduce and manage your stress through deep breathing, keeping fit emotionally, and getting sufficient sleep.

Deep Breathing

Breathing? That doesn't seem too complicated. We breathe all day and all night, but we gain weight nonetheless, so how is breathing going to help us? Well, there is a difference between breathing and deep breathing. What deep breathing is going to allow you to do is quickly and naturally calm your mind and body when you're faced with stressful experiences and self-limiting beliefs. When you take a minute to simply focus on breathing deeply and nothing else, it will allow you to clear your mind and shed the physical and mental stresses that you've accumulated.

So the first step toward setting yourself on the path to success is a deep breathing exercise that I call the one-minute mental tune-up. This exercise will help you relax and put you in the right frame of mind to move forward. Let's do that right now.

Begin by taking a slow, long, deep breath through the nostrils, filling your lungs to capacity with air. Hold that breath for a moment. Now begin to exhale slowly through your mouth as you mentally count backward from five . . . four . . . three . . . two . . . one. On the count of one, release all the rest of the air from your lungs and begin to take another long, slow breath through the nostrils, again filling your lungs to capacity. Again, hold your breath for a moment. And again, let some out slowly while you count backward. Five . . . four . . . three . . . two . . . one. When you get to one, let the remaining air out of your lungs again. Now take one last long, slow breath through your nostrils and hold it for a moment. Once more, let it out slowly as you count down. Five . . . four . . . three . . . two . . . one. When you reach one, this time, begin to breathe normally.

That's it. By repeating the deep breathing process in a controlled and focused manner three times, you will allow more oxygen to enter your bloodstream, calming your body and therefore your mind. You can change your mood in one minute simply by practicing this deep breathing exercise.

Deep breathing is a crucial skill that will allow you to reduce your stress and meditate by yourself. Whether you decide to use a guided meditation recording or soft music in a quiet, dimly lit room, deep breathing will allow you to transition easily from a state of mental and physical tension and stress to calmness.

Another complementary technique that can aid in achieving a serene state that will allow you to move forward with confidence is to repeat the word "calm" in your mind for thirty seconds while practicing deep breathing. This will help you to push all thoughts of food and stress aside, putting you in a proper state of mind to move forward.

Keeping Fit Emotionally

Your physical and mental well-being are very closely related. When you're feeling good physically, you feel good emotionally; when you're in a good place emotionally, you feel better physically and are more motivated to work yourself into better physical condition. Both physical and mental health can be achieved through a healthy lifestyle, not just, for example, eating well or quitting smoking but living well.

When you don't live well, you're only creating problems for yourself. If you live poorly, taking inadequate care of yourself to the point that you're often feeling pain or discomfort, you will feel miserable. If you're stressed out, sleeping poorly, working too much, worrying too much about work or family or money, and so on, it's going to make you feel physically fatigued and discomfited. It turns into a vicious cycle; once you get into a pattern in which you feel bad physically, it feeds into feeling bad mentally, which feeds into continuing to not care for yourself physically.

It's time to break the cycle.

Now that you have a goal in mind of achieving overall health, it's time to take the first step forward. You may already have given thought to your stressors before, but dig a little deeper now. Examine how you live. Pay particular attention to your reactions when faced with stress-inducing situations, and use the lessons learned from those situations to consciously alter your behavior in ways that will lessen the physical and mental stresses that you have to face. Try some of the following:

- Know your strengths and weaknesses and play to them. Get involved with activities and work that make you feel comfortable. Avoid unpleasant things of all sorts whenever possible.
- Do work that makes you feel appreciated, where you feel like you're accomplishing something, where you feel capable, and most importantly, where you enjoy yourself.

- Try to do something nice for someone else once every day.
- Don't always have to have the final word. You don't need to always show yourself that you're right.
- Put ideas, events, and even deadlines in a positive light; for example, "I would prefer to finish this job soon" rather than "I must get this job done."
- Take things one at a time. Don't start another task until you've finished the one before.
- Do your tasks the right way: make a list, prioritize, take time off in between, learn from your mistakes, and don't feel guilty or stressed if you don't finish as much as you planned.

You can only make changes successfully when you become willing, both consciously and subconsciously, to initiate them. Once you've reached the point at which you're dissatisfied with your weight and realize how it's impacting your physical and mental health, ruining your day-to-day life, you can't let it continue. You must become proactive to make the necessary changes to make your life long and enjoyable.

You don't have to start all at once either. Take things one at a time; transition into the diet. The more extreme the changes you think you have to make, the less inclined you're going to be to make them, so keep things simple. Think of it in terms of going swimming in the ocean early in the summertime. Some people are fine with just jumping on into the cold water, while others are more comfortable with getting their feet wet first then slowly wading further into the water, getting their body accustomed to the temperature before they fully commit themselves to the sea.

Decide which approach is right for you and start making changes in your life. If you feel good about just jumping right in, that's exactly what you should do. But if, like many people, you think that you might be better served by methodically taking minor steps and making changes a little at a time, the advice you're going to find below will help you still achieve your weight loss.

One easy way to begin is simply paying attention to labels and nutrition information. Start counting, just casually, how many grams of fat and carbohydrates you're eating every meal, keeping in mind that the goal is to keep your daily intake under 15 and 150. Just watch how your fat and carbs pile up, way over those marks, and now that you've started noticing how unhealthy so many of the foods you're eating are, begin cutting back steadily. This diet, like any, will only help you if you can stick to it, and you'll only be able to stick to it if you make the transition easy on yourself, so don't try to do too much too fast.

So since you don't want to rush yourself, start by just cutting out the big things. You'll find that a lot of single meals have more than 15 g of fat in them! But many foods, be they home prepared, frozen, or from a restaurant, have reasonable, tasty low-fat alternatives like the recipes in the back of this book. Start by picking out a few that sound tasty and cooking them up for dinner instead of, for example, ordering a pizza or picking up fast food. You may be surprised at just how good the lower-fat, lower-carb foods can be, and you'll feel a sense of accomplishment at having done something active and productive, making something with your own two hands that both tastes good and is good for you.

You can go along like this for a couple of weeks until you really have an understanding of what you're putting into your body and you've identified some recipes you like and have learned to repeat. Then once you're ready, set a date, and when that date comes, use the fat-and-carb counting habits you've gained to really make an adjustment and start eating better with some structure. Introducing structure to your diet is one of the biggest changes you'll make.

Putting a cap of any sort on your food intake is going to really help you get to the right place. Again, take it slow; there's no need to be overly ambitious and give yourself more than you can handle. If 15 and 150 is too much and too fast, then set an easier mark, say, 25 and 200. As long as you're moderating your intake, that's a great start. So practice 25 and 200 for a while if you need to and set a date a couple of weeks into it to take the next step and bring your intake down to 15 and 150.

Chapter 6

How to Eat

You may have heard before that how you eat is just as important as what you eat. But that statement has very little meaning without a proper understanding of what defines eating practices and bad eating habits. You will find that when you're trying to lose weight, having healthy, pro-weight loss eating practices will be just as important as the content of your meals and snacks. After all, it's difficult to constantly concentrate on eating right *all* the time; there are times in our lives when we simply have too much going on to keep count.

Although it's important to make those times the exception rather than the rule, we must be realists and acknowledge that they will indeed occur. If you form good eating habits, you can keep those occasions from affecting the progression of your weight loss. Just as importantly, with proper eating habits, you will put your body in the correct metabolic state to process what you eat efficiently so that all your hard work pays off and you lose weight.

With that in mind, let's define our terms. You already know that the way to lose weight is to stick with the 15/150 plan—no more than 15 g of fat and no more than 150 g of carbohydrates on a daily basis. But of course, not all fats and carbohydrates are created equal, as you can see by looking at any nutrition label. A label normally lists total fat on it, followed by several subcategories, including things such as saturated fat, trans fat, polyunsaturated fat, and monounsaturated fat. Similarly, under total carbohydrates, you might see the subcategories sugars, dietary fiber, and other carbohydrates.

Nutrition Facts

Serving Size 8 oz (227 g/8 oz)
Servings Per Container About 3

Amount Per Serving

Calories 130   Calories from Fat 0

% Daily Value*

Total Fat 0g	**0**%
Saturated Fat 0g	**0**%
Trans Fat 0g	
Cholesterol 0mg	**0**%
Sodium 95mg	**4**%
Total Carbohydrate 27g	**9**%
Dietary Fiber 5g	**21**%
Sugars 13g	
Protein 8g	

Vitamin A 130%	•	Vitamin C 110%	
Calcium 10%	•	Iron 6%	

---

* Percent Daily Values are based on a 2,000 calorie diet. Your daily values may be higher or lower depending on your calorie needs.

		Calories	2,000	2,500
Total Fat	Less than		65g	80g
Sat Fat	Less than		20g	25g
Cholesterol	Less than		300mg	300mg
Sodium	Less than		2,400mg	2,400mg
Total Carbohydrate			300g	375g
Dietary Fiber			25g	30g

Calories per gram:
   Fat 9 • Carbohydrate 4 • Protein 4

Nutrition labels are very easy to read! Highlighted here are the three areas of the label to focus on the most for the purposes of the 15/150 diet. While the other information is certainly also important to your overall health, these are the areas we're really concentrating on.

Serving Size: Nutritional information can be deceiving because one manufacturer may list one serving size, and another one may list a smaller serving size, making it look like their product contains less fat and carbs when in fact it might have more.

Total Fat, Saturated Fat and Trans Fat: Total fat is the one you'll be paying the most attention to, but whenever possible, avoid foods rich in saturated or trans fats.

Total Carbohydrate: While it's good to prioritize foods that have lower sugar, the overall carbs number is the one to use for your weight-loss goals.

Let's start with fat. Total fat is what you're going to count, but that doesn't mean you should ignore the others, as they can have a major impact on your health. Trans fats, which include both monounsaturated and polyunsaturated fats, have a major correlation to heart disease, as they serve to raise bad cholesterol, what's called LDL, and lower good cholesterol, HDL. Trans fat-containing foods are also inflammatory foods, so they can cause inflammation, or if you're suffering from inflammation already, eating more trans-fatty foods will make it worse.[2] That comfort food might not be so comforting after all. The U.S. Department of Agriculture's (USDA) *Dietary Guidelines for Americans 2005* advises that you keep your trans fat intake as low as possible due to the risk of heart disease.[3]

Saturated fat is also bad for your health in large quantities and can be present in such quantities in many popular foods, such as chocolate, dairy products, prepared foods, and red meat, including pork. High consumption of saturated fat has been linked to heart disease and cancer, and as such, the USDA's recommendation has been that Americans should severely cut their intake of saturated fat.

Ideally, of your fifteen allotted grams of fat daily, no more than three to four grams should be saturated fat, and none at all should be trans fats. You don't have to keep count of your saturated fat and trans fat intake like you keep count of 15 and 150 since eating no more than 15 g of fat a day will naturally keep those dangerous fats relatively low. It's simply something to be aware of.

Carbohydrates are a bit simpler. Again, as with fat, total carbohydrates are the ones to count, but there are some types of carbs that should be eaten more often and others that should be eaten less often. It's important to your health to eat the right carbohydrates; you're allowed 150 g a day, but there's no reason to waste them on unhealthy sugars. Dietary fiber is among the non-sugar carbohydrates that you'll frequently find

---

[2.] "Trans fat is double trouble for your heart health." *http://www.mayoclinic.com/health/trans-fat/CL00032.*

[3.] "Chapter 6: Fats." *http://www.health.gov/dietaryguidelines/dga2005/document/html/chapter6.htm.*

on nutrition labels. The USDA had this to say about dietary fiber in the *Dietary Guidelines for Americans 2005*:

> Diets rich in dietary fiber have been shown to have a number of beneficial effects, including decreased risk of coronary heart disease and improvement in laxation. There is also interest in the potential relationship between diets containing fiber-rich foods and lower risk of type 2 diabetes.[4]

As mentioned earlier, many labels list "other carbohydrates." These are typically what are considered "complex carbohydrates." These typically are carbohydrates found in fruits, vegetables, and whole grains and should be consumed with confidence within the boundaries of your diet.

The final carbohydrate to watch is, of course, sugar. Sugars can give you energy but are among the biggest culprits in weight gain. When you eat sugars, your body absorbs them into your bloodstream very quickly. Your body reacts to elevated blood sugar levels by creating more of the hormone insulin, which brings your blood sugar down when it's too high. It does this by removing the sugar from your blood and storing it in your tissue, effectively putting the weight on your body. Meanwhile, you gain no nutrients from sugar, hence why sugary foods are often noted for containing *empty calories*.

Many sugary foods also contain high-fructose corn syrup, which has been linked to diabetes and liver disease and has been found to contain mercury due to certain manufacturing processes. High-fructose corn syrup intake should be severely moderated; whenever you have sweetened foods or drinks, try to make sure that they're sweetened with natural sugar or no-calorie sugar substitutes. Again, sticking to eating no more than 150 g of carbs per day will automatically help you moderate your intake of high-fructose corn syrup, as most foods that contain it tend to be so high in carbs you won't be able to fit them into your diet.

Try to find foods you like that are low on the glycemic index. This index measures carbohydrates' effects on your blood sugar; foods that are lower

---

4.   "Chapter 7: Carbohydrates." *http://www.health.gov/dietaryguidelines/dga2005/ document/html/chapter7.htm*.

on the index break down slower, releasing glucose into your system at a moderate rate. Eating foods that are lower on the glycemic index will help you avoid diabetes and heart disease while also aiding in your weight-loss efforts. The Glycemic Index Foundation (http://*www.glycemicindex.com*) has a comprehensive database of foods and their place on the glycemic index; go on their Web site and look up some of your favorite foods to see how you're doing and what you can change.

In that vein, there are several easy-to-make dietary alterations that will both make it easier for you to follow the 15/150 diet and help you engage in healthy, anti-inflammatory eating to avoid the ill effects of these bad foods. For example, replace white potatoes with yams, white rice with wild rice or brown rice, and white breads and pastas with whole-grain breads and pastas. If you choose foods that are made with whole grains, your diet will automatically be improved in several respects. Whole grain foods tend to be less likely to contain high-fructose corn syrup or other dangerous additives. They also contain valuable antioxidants, vitamins, and minerals and are lower in fat and simple carbohydrates than refined grains. For that reason, your blood sugar will be more stable, which will keep you from gaining weight, your blood pressure will be lower, and you'll be more heart-healthy. Whole grains also are, of course, a valuable source of dietary fiber and other complex carbohydrates. Additionally, eating whole grains makes you feel more satiated for longer periods of time, making them a great weapon in your weight-loss arsenal.

What precisely is included under whole grains? They include barley, millet, brown rice, wild rice, buckwheat, oatmeal, and popcorn (eat it air-popped only for a high-fiber, low-fat, sugar-free snack!), as well as whole-wheat breads, pastas, cookies, and crackers.

Whole-grain foods really do taste naturally delicious, but if you're used to the taste of white bread, for example, the transition to whole-grain bread can be somewhat difficult; after all, food companies have spent decades getting us hooked on the less-healthy refined grains, high-fructose corn syrup, and so on because they're simply more profitable. It's going to take time to break out of those habits. Start by finding yourself a good whole-grain cereal to eat in the morning; if you need some more flavor than you might find in a typical multigrain cereal, find one that contains fruit or some other flavoring that will make it tastier to you. As with everything else, make the transition easy on yourself.

There are some other great habits that can be integrated into any successful dieter's routine. Some of these may work for you, and some may not. Find the ones that work for you. You might find them on this list, or you very well might come up with them on your own. As long as they help you lose weight and feel good about yourself and what you're doing, commit to them. Some of these are small changes that you should be able to make easily, while others are bigger and might be more difficult to make. As with the adaptation to 15 and 150, don't push yourself into doing everything at once if it's too much; you'll find things much more manageable if you make this a transition rather than a shock to the system.

Start with a small change. Drink a glass of water before every meal. Now, drinking water won't make you lose weight, but it does have several very positive health effects. For one, it replaces unhealthy sodas, alcoholic drinks, or juice cocktails with something that contains no fat, carbs, or calories—a quick and easy way to cut your intake. Moreover, drinking a glass of water before you eat makes you feel fuller, aiding in portion control.

It's important here to take a moment to elucidate the importance of portion control, as it may well be the single most important aspect of successfully dieting. To meet your goals of no more than 15 g of fat and 150 g of carbohydrates, you have to know the serving sizes of what you're eating and always you have to count each serving you consume. After all, the fat in the tasty treat with 2 g per serving and five servings per bag sure does add up if you eat the whole bag!

Drinking plenty of water (or other low-caloric drinks) will help you control your portions, but willpower is your strongest weapon here. Keep count of your fat and carbs with every serving you eat, and if you're getting toward those marks where you can't eat anymore, just stop for a moment and practice the deep breathing exercise from earlier in this chapter. Calm yourself and put things in perspective. Ask yourself one simple question: on a scale of 1 to 10, how full am I? If you are at a 6 or below, enjoy some more of your meal.

If you're at more like a 7 or higher, it's time to ease off. Wrap your plate, and save the rest of your meal for another time when you're actually hungry. It's still yours; it's not going anywhere. You can still have it later. No one is telling you not to eat it; just enjoy your leftovers at a later time or for lunch the next day. It will be a treat you can look forward to.

If you can't get into the habit of drinking water, have a cup of tea or perhaps Vitamin Water or other flavored waters. Make sure to count the carbs though, as some flavored waters have added sugar. Carbonated waters with flavor added can be a good thing as well, as the carbonation adds a little bit of bite to the flavor. Even diet soda works, although soda in general is not particularly healthy, so don't overdo it.

Many people find that they're able to control their portions, but because they're not eating as much as they're used to, they end up having a lot of between-meal snacks. A tall glass of water or flavored water, if you prefer, can help curb your appetite if you get hungry between meals. If that's not enough, have a very small amount of the food you're craving, along with a big glass of water. As with the other changes you're making, this can be a gradual one; have that little bit of food you crave but slowly reduce it until a glass of water alone will soothe your hunger.

Some people, especially those who are more active, need to eat every few hours rather than the normally accepted three meals a day. If you need a snack, one of the smaller recipes in the back of this book can satisfy your hunger while keeping you within the day's count. For example, the vanilla smoothie has just seven carbs and no fat, making it easy to fit into your diet any time of day! You never have to feel like you're depriving yourself of food on this diet; all you have to do is find low-fat, low-carb foods that you like, and with more and more companies realizing that healthier food is better for business, it's only going to get easier to find them. When you get to Bobbie's section, that's really going to help you fit the diet to your personal tastes.

People who overeat regularly can stretch out their stomachs; it's going to take time for your stomach to bounce back to its natural size. Stomach expansion is part of why it's so difficult to lose weight; once you're used to eating a lot of food, your body always desires a lot of food, and it takes time to condition yourself to feel otherwise. So naturally, one of the most important practices for you to get into is never, ever stuffing yourself. Halfway through your meal, ask yourself how full you are on a scale from 1 to 10; you know what to do from there.

If you fill your stomach up, it will expand to fit more, and that's not going to help your weight loss. You may have heard of or know someone who has gotten laparoscopic gastric band surgery, which essentially involves surgically placing a band around the top of your stomach that squeezes it so that you become physically incapable of overeating. It's an effective method, but surgery is dangerous, expensive, and unpleasant, with potential for complications and generally ruining the eating experience for you. It's certainly not an easy way out, especially because most people love food and don't want to have a semi-permanent limit on how much of it they can eat.

The techniques outlined in this book will help you go about things the natural way, using your self-control to eat right—a much more desirable option in terms of your long-term physical health.

Drinking water (and other low-calorie beverages) and counting each portion of food you enjoy are easy and effective weight-loss strategies, but they're just the beginning.

It's certainly true that some of the best-tasting foods are also some of the least healthy foods, but some healthy foods are among the best-tasting ones as well, such as the multigrain foods discussed earlier. One of the great keys to dieting success is finding healthy foods that you enjoy hence the recipes in this book, which Bobbie and I came up with to provide you with specific, delicious, low-fat, low-carb foods that you can integrate into your daily diet.

There are, of course, some foods that aren't going to work with the 15/150 diet. While you're trying to lose weight, you're going to have to almost entirely avoid red meat except as an occasional treat. Even the leanest beef can be difficult to fit into your 15 g fat allotment. If you must eat steak—and, again, do so rarely—cut as much of the fat from it as you can and lean toward small portions. Eating a lean 4 oz. steak doesn't sound like much when you're used to a 21 oz. porterhouse, but if you can't live without red meat in your diet, portion control is vital. Try to stay away from eating four-legged animals in general. If you can afford it, even as an occasional treat, ostrich is a wonderful alternative to beef. Ostrich filet looks and tastes like filet mignon but has about one-third of the fat!

Once you've lost enough weight and moved on the maintenance portion of the diet, you should be able to fit some more sizeable steaks into your diet, but if you want to lose weight, you do have to make some minor sacrifices, and that means that the big-time fatty red-meat-based foods—cheese-steaks, burgers, lamb chops, and so on—have to get left out until you get to the point where your body is back at its proper weight and you feel good enough about yourself to eat them. Americans tend to eat too much red meat as it is, and that can be a long-term health problem for reasons besides weight gain due to its content of saturated fat and cholesterol.

There are plenty of options for you to eat instead of red meat. Chicken, turkey, seafood, and beans are all excellent options that are lower in fat and carbs than beef and other red meats and can be prepared similarly to great effect. And you will find that eating these foods rather than red meat will help you have healthier eating habits.

Eating red meat is not just a bad eating habit, but it's also one that can lead to even worse eating habits. When you cut those hamburgers and steak sandwiches out of your life, you are going to have that many fewer opportunities to eat the foods that usually come with them—french fries, fried onion rings, and so on. These massively unhealthy foods often come with your burger in very large quantities and contain huge amounts of fat and especially saturated fat. You're better off without them. So when you go out to a restaurant and you don't order a hamburger—maybe you get a low-fat, grilled entrée instead—you're more likely to get a soup or a salad rather than a plate full of fries.

On that note, we come to restaurant eating. Eating out can be, but doesn't have to be, one of the biggest threats to your weight-loss efforts. The food at restaurants is delicious but often lacks the detailed nutrition information that you need to monitor your fat and carbohydrate intake and frequently is doused in thick, rich sauces that are surprisingly high in fat, among other "hidden" dangers. Eating at a restaurant also tempts you with appetizers and desserts to go with your entrée, creating the risk of becoming overfilled as well as simply eating too much fat and carbs.

For example, half a cup of alfredo sauce is good for about nine grams of fat, including two grams of saturated fat. That's half a cup. Order a nice, large-portioned fettuccine alfredo at an Italian restaurant and you could easily find twice that amount of sauce in your dish. A simple pasta dish and it already puts you over the day's limit for fat intake. Cheesy sauces, such as alfredo, as well as hollandaise sauce, béarnaise sauce, and gravies are very high in fat and easy to eat a lot of without even realizing.

In general, when ordering food that comes with sauce at a restaurant, try to order your entrée grilled with the sauce on the side so you can control your intake, adding enough sauce to get the taste without eating extra fat to stay within the 15/150 diet.

The same goes for salad dressings. In fact, salad in general is one of the more dangerous foods you can order at a restaurant because you might think, since you're ordering a salad, that you're eating healthy. This in turn can make you figure that you can sneak a cheeseburger in the next day because you just ate a salad the day before, and that will offset it. Well, when that salad is loaded up with croutons, cheese, nuts, and sometimes meat, along with being doused in dressing, you'll find that it's not so healthy after all! Two tablespoons of Caesar dressing (the typical serving), for example, contain a whopping nine grams of fat—and if you get dressing put on your salad at a restaurant, they're not about to measure out two tablespoons. That's not even counting all the fat and carbs from the croutons, cheeses, nuts, and meats, which also need to be tracked.

With all that considered, you should strongly consider ordering your food with sauce on the side or bringing your own sauces and dressings. Many restaurants can provide fat-free or low-fat dressing for your salad. If you're at a restaurant and they don't have a low-fat dressing you like, ask for balsamic vinegar and Dijon mustard, mix the two together, and voila'—your own fat-free salad dressing! This is a good option if you're against bringing your own sauces and salad dressings along with you to restaurants. Although it's understandable that you might feel self-conscious bringing containers of sauce or dressing to a restaurant with you, compare that feeling to how happy you're going to be when you have to go out and buy new clothes for all the weight you've lost!

The great thing about bringing your own sauces and dressings is that you not only know the fat and carb content of your foods, but also you can control your own portions, allowing you to keep an accurate count for the day. Experiment with making your own salad dressings; lemon juice, balsamic vinegar, and buttermilk dressing are good, healthy options. Find low-fat, low-carb sauces in the store that you like and bring those along as well. There's no shame in wanting to eat healthy even if you're out at a restaurant.

While you're eating out, you may get vegetables served along with your meal. These vegetables are often stir-fried or grilled, sometimes with sauces, offsetting the positive effects of the vitamins and the nutrients within. When you order dishes with cooked vegetables, ask for them to be steamed rather than the cooking process the restaurant would otherwise use. Steamed vegetables without any butter or sauce added retain their nutrient content better than grilled or fried vegetables while not adding any fat or carbohydrates to the vegetables' natural contents. Of course, vegetables are a valuable part of any dieter's food arsenal, particularly when you're out to eat; the more veggies you eat, the less you can fill up on bread and meat.

One final thing to look out for when eating at a restaurant is all the food you can eat before or after your main course. Since you're counting carbs, avoid the bread. Appetizers and desserts are the biggest risks here. They're so tempting and so rarely healthy. Under appetizers, we find many fried or cheesy foods—full of fat! If you want an appetizer, order a shrimp or crab cocktail or have fresh clams or oysters plain (not casino—or Rockefeller style).

Meanwhile, under desserts, we find chocolate cake, cheesecake, ice cream, crème brûlée, bread pudding, and so on. Unless the restaurant happens to have some explicitly healthy desserts that you can fit into your diet, wait to eat your post meal sweets until you get home and can have a treat that you know will fit into your daily count.

Another helpful hint: if you're out to eat with someone who isn't dieting, share a little bit of their dessert. And we mean a little bit. If you only eat a spoonful, just to get a taste, you will feel less deprived.

CHAPTER 7
EXERCISE AND MAINTENANCE

Strictly speaking, this is not a diet-and-exercise plan, but there are some basic things that all people should do to remain in good health. Our bodies weren't made to sit around all day and do nothing; we need to keep the muscles working. This doesn't need to happen at the gym necessarily, although it's certainly recommended that you go to the gym. But even if not, our bodies need to get a chance to move around. It can be all too easy to put on weight if you work in an office every day and have to sit at a desk from 9 to 5, but no matter what your job, you should get up and move around at least a little bit every day. It will make you feel better physically, and as noted before, when you're in better shape physically, you're going to have stronger mental health as well.

According to the American Heart Association (AHA), cardiovascular disease is the # 1 cause of death in America. Cardiovascular disease happens for a lot of reasons that you can control—poor diet habits, smoking, and a lack of exercise. The AHA has some simple suggestions that will both help you avoid cardiovascular disease and get your muscles enough work on a day-to-day basis that they stay strong and fit.

Even low-to-moderate intensity activities, when done for as little as thirty minutes a day, bring benefits. These activities include pleasure walking, climbing stairs, gardening, yard work, moderate-to-heavy housework, dancing and home exercise.

More vigorous aerobic activities, such as brisk walking, running, swimming, bicycling, roller skating and jumping rope are best for improving the fitness of the heart and lungs.[5]

One thing I have done personally is buy a pedometer. I highly recommend pedometer ownership to all my patients—those who need to lose weight and those who don't. They're inexpensive—you can pick up a decent one for $15 or so—and will prove invaluable to your weight-loss and weight-maintenance efforts. My pedometer allows me to keep track of how many steps I take every day, with a goal of taking a minimum of 5,000 steps every day. And I do; I count 225 steps each way from my parking spot up the stairs to my second-floor office. The hallway in my office, which I'm always walking up and down to go get things or pacing while on the phone, is 55 steps each way. It takes 425 steps to walk to the drugstore across the street to grab a drink and a snack and 425 steps back. It's about 650 steps to walk over to the nearby eatery and grab a sandwich for lunch. My dentist's office is just around the corner; it takes 1,100 steps to walk over there twice a year for regular teeth cleaning. My podiatrist's office is down the street at 1,175 steps.

In an average day at the office, from parking my car in the morning to getting back into it in the evening, I take 3,900 to 4,200 steps. That's not counting walking my dogs in the morning before I leave for the office and then again once I get home, depending on how much they want to trot about—that can easily be significantly more than 1,000 steps per trip. In fact, if you have the time, money, and patience to get a dog, I highly recommend it; the companionship and the exercise from walking and playing alone make it more than worthwhile, and if you don't have time to housebreak a puppy, your local shelters are sure to have housebroken adult dogs that have been given up.

If you eat right, that is, follow the 15/150 diet or the modified version of it for weight maintenance that's covered in this chapter, and take 5,000 steps every day, you'll never gain weight. If you eat right and always take 10,000 steps a day, the weight will melt off your body. Walking 5,000

---

5.   Physical Activity and Cardiovascular Health Fact Sheet, *http://americanheart.org/ presenter.jhtml?identifier=820*.

steps is roughly equivalent, depending on the length of your stride, to 2.5 miles a day. That may sound like a lot, but it's not too difficult to look for ways to walk places rather than driving, and if you do that regularly, you'll be surprised how quickly the steps can add up. Since you're going to be wearing the pedometer, make something of a game of it—your goal is to get to 5,000 to "win" every single day, so sneak in each and every extra step you possibly can.

Besides helping to prevent disease, getting regular cardiovascular work will stimulate your metabolism, which will help you lose weight. The goal of most of what we've outlined in this book is to get your metabolism back to working for you; reducing your stress, getting sufficient exercise, and eating right are all key components of putting yourself in the most efficient metabolic state possible.

Regular exercise retains its importance once you've successfully lost all that extra weight as well. No diet ever really ends; if you go off a diet and slip back into the same bad eating habits from before, all that weight will come right back. So it's key to continue with the same simple exercises—walking, taking the stairs, and so on. Stay active and continue with a version of the 15/150 guidelines that's modified to fit the foods you want to eat.

Quite a few of my patients have found that simply slightly raising the fat and carb counts to 20 and 200 allowed them to maintain their weight loss. If that works for you and you don't gain weight at 20/200, then that's a great place to stick at for the rest of your life. But the great thing about maintaining your weight loss on the 15/150 diet is its flexibility. If you'd like to eat more bread and other carbohydrates, then by all means, eat even more than 200 carbs, but cut your fat intake proportionately so that you don't gain weight. Or perhaps, now that you've lost weight, you'd like to get back to eating some red meat and other fatty yet delicious items. That's no problem; you can easily eat up to 30 g of fat in a day but cut the carbohydrates down proportionately. It's pretty easy to work with; just keep your life in balance. If you eat more carbs, compensate by eating less fat, and if you eat more fat, eat fewer carbs. Simple!

Remember though that this is strictly for the maintenance portion of the diet. Although this is certainly a good rule to remember for purposes of compensation if you slip up and eat too much fat or too many carbs one day, it's not something that should be applied to your day-to-day weight-loss efforts. Once you've achieved your weight-loss goal, you'll be able to afford the occasional slipup, and even if you feel you have the requisite self-control, follow the adjusted guidelines in a pretty general sense by not necessarily counting every day but still paying close attention to your intake. But for purposes of weight loss, you should stick to 15 g of fat and 150 carbs, as it's the simplest plan possible; doing otherwise has too much potential to cause confusion and make you lose track of your progress throughout the day.

Never be discouraged and never get stressed out if you slip up! Once you've lost that extra weight, the hard part will be over. As long as you remain reasonably active and committed to keeping track of your food intake, you will never have a problem with gaining that weight back.

At this point, this book makes a transition from the theoretical to the practical as I turn it over to Bobbie Freiberg, a patient of mine who successfully lost a lot of weight on the 15/150 diet. Before she came to me, Bobbie was just like you—dissatisfied with her weight and dissatisfied with the many diets out there but still ready and willing to commit to a healthy lifestyle that would let her lose weight and keep it off. From her, you will learn more specifics about what to eat, what not to eat, and generally, how to live the 15/150 lifestyle. She has also come up with simple, original recipes that have helped her in her weight-loss journey and will give you ideas for your own snacks and meals. Keep going!

CHAPTER 8
ANOTHER INTRODUCTION

In the first half of this book, you learned the technical side of the 15/150 diet. Now it's time for the practical side. It's time to learn how to eat well while losing weight and keeping it off. I'm going to show you how to tweak the way you cook, shop, and order out so that you can bring out the slimmer you.

My name is Bobbie. I am in my early fifties and, like many others, gradually put on extra pounds over the years. When I looked in the mirror, I still saw the beautiful maiden I was in my mid-twenties. I couldn't understand why my clothes kept getting tighter and tighter. Were they shrinking in my closet due to my heater? Did I leave them too long in the dryer? Did the dry cleaners give me the wrong pants?

I had a more million excuses, but the camera doesn't lie! This heavy woman kept appearing in our family photos. I know the camera can put on an extra ten pounds, but this was way more than ten! I would crop off an arm, half my body—whatever made me appear thinner in the pictures—but some photos I just couldn't fix. I didn't know that person in the photos, and I knew I had to get back to the old me.

I've tried many diets over the years, only to be stuck on a rollercoaster. You know how it goes—lose two pounds, then gain three. Like many others, I tried counting calories and points, eating certain foods, eliminating certain foods, eating extra fiber, and exercising more. I even thought about buying every diet I saw on late-night infomercials. My problem was that, like many others, I like quantity as much as quality. It's hard to give up my sweets, salts, and grown-up drinks. In short, I wanted a miracle diet. And I found it.

One day, about a year before I started on this book, I was shopping and ran into a friend I had not seen in months. As I went to get her attention, I realized that I wasn't even sure that was her. This woman had just lost fifty pounds in less than six months! I complimented her profusely and asked her how she lost the weight. She told me about the 15/150 diet. She explained how easy it was and that she didn't even feel like she was dieting! She was in the store to buy new pants because her old ones were falling off! She gave me Dr. Steven Rosenberg's number, and on that day, my weight-loss journey began.

The problem with dieting is that I absolutely love to eat! I've got a sweet tooth, a salty tooth, a savory tooth—you name it. I love to eat all kinds of food, and I don't like to go hungry. I have never had any lasting success with a diet that cut my food intake or forbid me too many foods. I also like martinis or glasses of wine with dinner and haven't given them up either! I didn't get surgery, buy any special pills or creams or packaged foods, go to meetings, feel deprived, or spend a fortune. If you've bought this book, you've already spent what you need to on this diet!

I lost forty-five pounds in less than seven months and have kept it off ever since. I never gave up the foods I love, like ice cream cones, chocolate muffins, and pumpkin pie, and I sure didn't give up my martinis!

So how did I do it? What did I eat? What are the dietary secrets to success? Read on and find out.

CHAPTER 9
BOBBIE'S STORY

I am not a strong-willed person. I can't just pick a diet and stick with it on my own. I need cheering, coaching, and positive feedback. So by my friend's suggestion, I went to see Dr. Steven Rosenberg. We met for an hour, discussed my eating habits, and found that my biggest problem was the hidden fat that I didn't realize I was eating. I would go out and get what I thought was a nice, healthy salad, not realizing that the dressing had over 60 g of fat! There goes my effort to lose weight!

Over the course of a thirty-minute relaxation session, Dr. Rosenberg taught me the 15/150 diet plan. He also told me the one thing I needed to hear: regardless of age, height, weight, gender, or lifestyle, the diet is the same for everyone. But more importantly, you are absolutely scientifically guaranteed to lose weight!

That's what kept me going when after I lost ten pounds in the first month, I plateaued for a couple of weeks. The entire time, I never felt like I was dieting, so I thought I might be doing something wrong. But I kept hearing Dr. Rosenberg's promise that I was guaranteed to lose weight, so I stuck with it, and after my body stopped fighting me, more pounds just peeled off and off, never to be seen again!

It's like riding a bike: once you get the hang of it, you can just take off! We're not going to just leave you stranded though; the healthy, low-fat, low-carb recipes in this book will provide you with many a meal, and you'll also be able to visit www.15-150diet.com for new recipes and extra encouragement!

We all need help. I'm kind of compulsive when it comes to food. As much as I want to be in control, the smell of pizza or freshly baked chocolate cake can seduce me into an eating frenzy! There are so many delicious yet fattening foods that it can be unbelievably hard to resist. That's why it will help you to practice the program in chapter 4. It will help ingrain the 15/150 diet plan in your mind and provide you the mental support that, if you're anything like me, will be crucial to staying the course.

The best part of the 15/150 diet is the results. Week after week, day after day, you will lose weight. Friends and even strangers have come up to me and told me how great I look now—always good for my self-esteem! A friend of mine who'd lost weight once told me that she knew she wouldn't gain it back since she loved the "feeling of being thin". Now I know what she means; it's so amazing to go into my closet and know my clothes will fit!

One of Dr. Rosenberg's patients e-mailed me this story, and it impressed me so much that I knew I had to find a place for it in this book. Not only did she succeed in losing weight, but also the diet had a positive impact on her family's health! So here is what Pam had to say about the diet:

I hate the word "diet"! It means I cannot have what I want. But that is not a problem anymore for me. I used to think I was a good eater but remained heavy since my first child was born twenty-five years ago. I found that eating low fat and low carb is easy. I am about eighteen pounds lighter now and have no intent of stopping! Here's the funny thing. My husband went to his cardiologist last week, and the doctor congratulated him on losing fifteen pounds and dropping his cholesterol. He wasn't even on the diet; he just ate what I did! When I went to my doctor, they were looking at my cholesterol from my last visit before I started this diet to possibly regulate me on cholesterol medication. When they rechecked my numbers, they said I didn't need any medication! I have not had a heartburn issue since I started the 15/150 diet! Frankly, this is one of the best decisions I have made, and I'm looking forward to starting my son on a low-fat, low-carb diet this summer. Thank you, Dr. Rosenberg, for showing me the way to help my family and myself!

CHAPTER 10
CUTTING FAT AND CARBOHYDRATES

You've already learned the basics of the diet. Each day, eat no more than 15 g of fat and no more than 150 g of carbohydrates. This is much easier than you might think! You don't have to count calories or points, so as long as you can find foods that fit the bill—and there are tons of them!—there's no limit on your food intake.

One thing that I discovered early on was that it's the subtle fat and carbs, the ones you don't expect, that really make you gain weight.

There are very simple solutions to cutting that sneaky fat out. The first thing I learned is to cook with the spray oils with zero fat. That doesn't hurt you in flavor. Then I started looking more actively and found low fat and no fat tomato sauces and marinades for cooking my vegetables and entrees. It's easy to have control in your own kitchen.

When eating out, I take a small container of fat-free dressing to restaurants and order my salad dry which really cut down my fat intake. I order my entree grilled with either the sauce on the side or perhaps salsa instead. If I'm in the mood for breakfast, I get an egg substitute omelet with vegetables and rye toast dry with a little jelly. You can easily ask for fruit or tomato slices instead of the hash browns. Lunch is easy. I get a turkey breast sandwich on rye bread, add mustard, tomatoes, onions and extra pickles! These are very healthy meals and extremely low in fat!

Reading food labels will help you tremendously! You can pick up one jar of sauce which contains ten grams of fat, where another sauce on the same shelf contains only one gram of fat. The best part is that they almost taste the same!

Another important thing to remember about labels is to check the serving size. Nutrition information on labels can be highly misleading due to making serving sizes smaller for labeling purposes than they are for eating purposes. So if that jar has a serving for six on it, you have to do your multiplication!

All the big supermarkets carry lots of healthy food options these days; they're just not as well-advertised or popular as the fattening foods we've all come to know and love. So when you go to the supermarket, treat it like a treasure hunt. Make a game out of shopping the first few times you go, searching for the tasty-looking alternatives with low fat and low carbs until you get the right products for your delicious meals. You can still have the dressing and the sauces that you love, but just choose the low-fat version, which tends to taste just the same, and your body will thank you.

Another fatty and delicious food to watch for is cheese. That's a tough one; everyone loves cheese. Unfortunately, most of it is still very high in fat. So what do you do? There are excellent nonfat mozzarella, cheddar, feta and American cheeses you can buy at almost any store. It's still real cheese, just made from skim milk; it still tastes great, and you can pretty much eat as much of it as you want. You can still mix cheese into every meal, from your morning eggs to sandwiches, soups, and toppings for grilled dishes and vegetables.

Instead of buying fresh eggs, which contain a lot of fat, you can buy 100 percent egg whites or egg substitutes. No fat, no carbs, and they're great for omelets, quiches, turkey meatloaf, pies, and many other dishes.

Red meat is something to avoid, but if you can make it through an entire day with zero fat, a broiled 6 oz. filet mignon for dinner is exactly fifteen grams, so treat yourself once in a while! For more everyday eating, lean turkey breast, chicken, ham, Canadian bacon, lean pork, and some veal are either low-fat or fat-free. Enjoy them. I always keep chicken breast or sliced turkey breast in my refrigerator. I count them as zero fat and zero carbs—part of my free menu that I can eat as much as I want to anytime! But if you want some veal, look up how it is prepared and keep track of those fat grams.

Many kinds of seafood are also excellent choices for avoiding fat intake, but just make sure they are prepared in a way that you can enjoy them without added fat from sauces or oils.

One of my favorite things to do is to tweak existing recipes, working in low-fat and low-carb ingredients. This is a huge part of how I managed to lose weight while not giving up my favorite foods. Here's a comparison of a standard cheesecake recipe and my alternative:

Regular Cheesecake	*Bobbie's Cheesecake*
8 oz. package of cream cheese	16 oz. fat-free cream cheese
8 oz. plain yogurt	6 oz. fat-free Greek yogurt
1 cup ricotta cheese	No ricotta
1/2 cup sugar and 1 tbsp. vanilla	2/3 cup sugar-free French vanilla syrup
1 egg	1/3 cup egg substitute
Pie crust	No pie crust

Combine all ingredients in a blender and mix thoroughly. Spray spring form pan with nonstick cooking spray; pour mixture in. Bake at 350 degrees for approximately one hour fifteen minutes, until the top starts to brown. Remove and let cool for one hour then refrigerate for three hours before serving.

My version is fat-free and has minimal carbs. Sprinkle with cinnamon and add fat-free whipped cream and/or fresh berries on top to vary your flavor. You can do the very same thing with most recipes. Just be creative; you may have to experiment a couple of times, but the treat and the weight loss are worth the effort!

The Fat Recap

- No more than fifteen grams per day.
- Avoid oils, nuts, eggs, regular cheese, and red meats.
- Enjoy lean turkey breast, chicken breast, Canadian bacon, lean pork, fish, and seafood.

- Find great versions of either low-fat, or fat free salad dressings, mayo, yogurt, sour cream, cream cheese and other cheeses, puddings, whipped cream, etc.
- You may have red meat if you want a very small portion, but make sure to count that fat!
- Use egg whites or egg substitutes.
- Use Butter Buds or butter-flavored cooking spray instead of real butter to get that buttery taste without any fat.

Carbohydrates, like fat, can be sneaky. You don't always think about eating them, but if you don't pay close attention to what you eat, it's easy to take in so many carbs that it's impossible to lose weight. So we're going to limit our carbs, not cut them out all together but keep it to no more than 150 grams per day.

The first step is to avoid the whites: bread, rice, potatoes, mayo, and pasta. Instead, pick up some whole grain bread and whole grain pasta. Instead of mashed potatoes, eat sweet potatoes (you can mash them too). Instead of white rice, eat brown and wild rice, which have plenty of health benefits in addition to having fewer carbs.

Fruit is good for you, but all fruits have carbs. Grapes (and raisins), cranberries, and cherries are all relatively high in carbs. So eat all kinds of fruit; it is part of a balanced diet after all, but moderate your intake and keep track. The appendix at the back of this book details fat and carb values for a wide variety of fruits. A simple "rule of thumb" that Dr. Rosenberg taught me was to count each serving of fruit, the size of an apple, as 20 carbs.

As far as alcohol goes, many wines are actually quite low in carbs, so you will often find that you have the leeway to indulge in your vintage of choice. Vodka and other distilled liquors are free (but not on your liver, so don't overdo it!), and you can add sugar-free syrups and flavorings or have it straight up with a lemon or lime. Beer is extremely high in carbs, so moderate your intake and count the carbs. But you can also find lower-carb beers!

The Carbohydrate Recap

- No more than 150 grams per day.
- Avoid white bread, white rice, potatoes, corn, soda, and sweet alcoholic drinks.
- Enjoy whole-grain bread, brown or wild rice, sweet potatoes and yams, and low carb-low fat drinks.
- Find versions of the foods you love (often different brands) without added sugar, especially high-fructose corn syrup.
- Count each fruit you eat.
- Vegetables are great, but make sure you count the carbs in the starchy ones like corn, beans, peas, potatoes, and rice.

CHAPTER 11
A DAY IN BOBBIE'S LIFE

Now let's get practical. After all, we can only list how you can eat one food and not eat another so much before it all means nothing to you. Let's go through a typical day in my life.

Like most other people, I've got to have my coffee first thing in the morning. I typically have about three cups to get properly wired for the day, and I drink it with fat-free creamer. Whole milk (or even 1 or 2 percent) tastes great, but if you replace it with fat-free creamer in your coffee, you'll be surprised at how rich your coffee tastes.

Ever since I entered middle age, my sleeping habits have become about as reliable as my internal thermostat. To translate, I never know when I'm going to get up. And when I do, I know that I have to get my exercise in before I shower for the day, or else I will find a hundred excuses not to do it.

I used to think that playing tennis was exercise. It may be for many people, but in reality, the way I move on the court does not burn calories. However, I have found something that I love and have been doing for over twenty years: walking.

I love to walk in the morning—quietly, at my own pace. My morning walk is a combination of mind therapy, exercise, and dog walking. I typically walk at my most comfortable fast pace for about three miles. If it's raining, I'll work my way to the gym and do some weight training. I understand this is something that I should be doing at my age, so I let the weather schedule my exercise routine.

Like most people who have had weight issues, I wish I could tell you that I was an avid exerciser, but I'm not—never was and never will be.

But the good news is that you don't need to be either! Just do the best you can. Try to realize when your energy level is at its peak and find an exercise routine that you enjoy. This will be your best chance of burning those extra, unwanted pounds and calories that you are trying to expel.

I have been walking and playing tennis for over twenty years but continued to gain weight all through that time. At first, I thought that there might be a medical condition, like menopause or a thyroid condition, that was keeping me from losing weight, but the reality was that I simply wasn't eating right. Only since I went on the 15/150 diet did I go from a size 12 to a size 6. I didn't change my exercise habits at all for this diet. The difference lies solely in the systematic reduction of carbs and fat.

Now, before I go for my walk, I do like a little something to eat. Of course, I don't always have the same level of hunger. Sometimes a piece of fruit will do; other times, something with my coffee, like a muffin or cookie. When I'm really hungry, I go for an omelet.

But maybe you want to know how a full day of eating might look on the 15/150 diet—after all, it's one thing to say that you want to cut your fat and carbs and another thing to find the right foods to do it. So here's a rough approximation of a real day of eating by a real person—me—who has really lost weight.

Breakfast

My favorite breakfast food is the omelet. Sound boring? Clearly you need to put more tasty things in your omelet. I use egg substitutes, nonfat mozzarella cheese, diced tomatoes, and oregano, with one or two slices of fat-free ham on the side. Cook your omelet up with nonfat cooking spray, not oil. This breakfast is almost entirely free, next to no fat and carbs at all! But if I know I'm hungry and I'm going to be good for the rest of the day, I'll add rye toast with fat-free cream cheese and jelly—add fifty carbs.

One thing I love to do for a snack is to combine fat-free ricotta cheese with sugar-free flavored syrups. It doesn't sound like much, but it comes out tasting like the inside of Italian cannoli, and it's got no fat and no carbs!

Lunch

When I am trying to be really good, I will make myself lettuce wraps instead of sandwiches. Pull a large leaf of lettuce and stuff it with turkey breast, leftover chicken, or fat-free ham and add fat-free mayo, some tomatoes, and onions or peppers and eat as many as you like. This meal is almost entirely free of fat and carbs, and it tastes great! If I skipped the morning toast, I can put it on whole-grain bread, a pita, or Jewish rye—just add about forty carbs.

Another thing I love is the fat-free potato chips. Add a few of them and just another twenty carbs and no fat!

Salads are wonderful, but watch those dressings! Also skip the pine nuts, cranberries, raisins, cheeses (unless you know they are fat-free), and sesame seeds when possible. These are high in either fat or carbs and create hidden dangers when you're trying to cut down. But go ahead and add fish, lean meat, or egg whites to your salad for protein.

Soups are great too, but just read the labels for fat and carbs. If you can make your own, go for it. I do add a couple of things. I may buy a tomato soup and melt fat-free mozzarella or cheddar cheese into the mix—delicious! Or for a great onion soup, I grill onions and mushrooms, add fat-free beef broth, and heat and melt fat-free mozzarella cheese. It's filling, tasty, and entirely free of fat and carbs!

Dinner

Obviously, a girl's got to have her martini. The wonderful thing about vodka is no fat and no carbs. Drink all the martinis you want within reason, but just stay away from beer unless you can afford the carbs!

I usually like to grill. You're limited in meat choices by the lack of red meat, but the great thing about chicken is that it's a blank canvas, and you can make it into anything you want. Grilled chicken breast with fat-free marinara sauce and fat-free mozzarella cheese makes a wonderful entrée! Add a salad and grilled or steamed veggies and you've got a delicious meal!

After Dinner

Since I've been good all day, it's time to reward myself with some tasty snacks, but I don't want to undo today's progress! Since I have a salty tooth as well as a sweet one, I got some multigrain pretzels (if you've never had them, you're missing out) to dip in mustard—three grams of fat and twenty-one carbs—no problem.

But then it's time to satisfy my sweet tooth, and I do that with a low-fat chocolate ice cream cone! Three grams of fat and twenty-eight carbs and I've been so good all day that I can have two and I'm still under 15 and 150.

If I'm still hungry for more, fat-free Jell-O with fat-free whipped cream is always a tasty snack, and I can have a glass of wine too!

Free (and Affordable) Foods

Think of food as a tool that you're using in your weight loss rather than an enemy you're avoiding. Find foods you like from this list and use them as staples in your everyday diet.

The Free:

- Egg omelets with fat-free cheddar, mozzarella, or American cheese: Add all the veggies and seasoning you'd like.
- Turkey breast: Use romaine lettuce and fat-free mayo to make lettuce rollups for lunch.
- Chicken breast: Grill with fresh-squeezed lemon and pepper and place on a bed of lettuce for a great salad.
- Tuna fish: Make a tuna salad with fat-free mayo, celery, onions, and some pickle juice and stuff it inside egg white halves or celery. (Keep in mind that you can make chicken salad, turkey salad, fat-free ham salad, egg salad, and salmon salad. I think you get the idea here.)
- Lettuces and veggies, including pickles and roasted peppers, with tzatziki (which has a couple of carbs in it, so do count those if you have a good amount).
- Fat-free ricotta cheese with sugar-free flavored syrups, with vanilla-flavored syrup—it tastes just like a cannoli! Experiment and see what tasty things you can come up with!

- Fat-free cheeses' can be used with the same versatility as regular cheeses. They're available in many grocery stores and can be ordered online.
- Salsa: This is great for fish toppings as well as a dip. Look in the recipe section for a fat-free refried bean dip with salsa—a wonderful surprise!
- Sugar-free Jell-O with fat-free whipped cream.
- Diet sodas, teas, and coffees.

The Affordable:

- Balsamic vinegar: Any well-aged (twelve years or more) balsamic will do just fine. It's a little more expensive but well worth it! (Younger balsamic is much more vinegary and less sweet.) I use it as a salad dressing or for cooking. I actually cooked scallops and mushrooms in it the other night and placed them over lettuce—out of this world! Oh, did I mention that for one tablespoon, there's zero fat and three grams of carbs? Not bad!
- Lox: Combine it with fat-free cream cheese or fat-free Greek yogurt. Try putting it on top of a cucumber slice and adding some scallions.
- Fat-free potato chips.
- Multigrain pretzels or chips.
- Fat-free refried bean dip.
- Low-fat popcorn and fat-free caramel popcorn.
- Wasabi peas. (Note: Spicy foods tend to kill your appetite!)
- Low-fat, sugar-free (or low-sugar) ice cream products.
- Low-fat, sugar-free (or low-sugar) muffins and cookies.
- Sugar-free and fat-free puddings.
- Fat-free yogurt, especially Greek yogurt. This is great for salad dressings, potato toppings, and my favorite is for the Yogurt Smoothie recipe!

There are lots of other great free and affordable foods in the recipes section, and of course you can always experiment with cooking on your own! More tasty and healthy foods will be posted on our website, and we look forward to posting your creations too!

Bon appétit! I hope you enjoy the recipes!

Chapter 12
Recipes

These recipes have all been developed explicitly to fit comfortably into a diet that allows for no more than 15 grams of fat and 150 grams of carbohydrates. They were also developed to feed not only the dieter but also the entire family, so they had to be not just healthy but tasty too! Finally, as you've already read, they were developed by someone who loves to eat but does not love to diet.

These recipes have passed the taste test with some of the pickiest eaters that we know, but if they don't fit into what you want to eat, by all means, try something different! Make your own recipes. Tweak these. Find others online, either on our website or elsewhere. This diet is flexible; make it work for you. The recipes that follow are just a start. All the fat and carb listings are per serving.

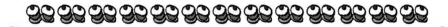

Bite-Sized Chocolate Cups

Ingredients

2 prepackaged dark Belgian chocolate cups
2 tbsp. fat-free whipped cream
2 slices of strawberry, mango, banana, or other fruit of choice

Directions

Fill each chocolate cup with fat-free whipped cream and add a slice
of your favorite fruit for a quick and easy dessert!

Serves: 1
Fat per serving: 4 g
Carbs per serving: 12 g

Asparagus Crab Soup

Ingredients

1 bunch fresh asparagus
32 oz. fat-free, low-sodium chicken broth
1 cup lump crabmeat
2 tbsp. shallots
1 tbsp. minced garlic
1/2 fresh lemon
8 oz. fat-free creamer or fat-free sour cream

Directions

Chop asparagus and cook in chicken broth. Once cooked to your liking, add sour cream (or fat-free creamer), crabmeat, shallots, and garlic and squeeze the fresh lemon into the soup. Serve hot or cold!

Servings: 6
Fat per serving: 0 g
Carbs per serving: 10 g

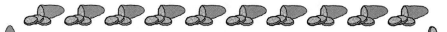

Chilled Cucumber Soup

Ingredients

3 large cucumbers
15 mint leaves (or dill and garlic if you prefer)
1/4 tbsp. fresh ginger powder
17 oz. fat-free Greek yogurt
Salt and pepper to taste
Optional: 3 oz. cup lump crabmeat or shrimp

Peel cucumbers, slice, and put in blender along with the other ingredients, except the optional crabmeat. Blend well, then add the crabmeat if desired and chill for 3 hours before serving.

This makes a wonderful, healthy treat for any time during the day!

Servings: 4
Fat: 0 g
Carbs: 6 g

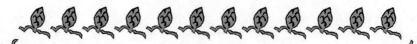

Stuffed Artichokes

Ingredients

32 oz. fat-free chicken broth
1/4 cup fat-free mozzarella cheese (also can substitute fat-free feta cheese)
4 large artichokes
Salt to taste
Optional: shrimp, sardines, ground chicken breast, and/or mushrooms

Directions

Clean artichokes by cutting off tips of leaves. Place in pot with the chicken broth, and cook for approximately 40 minutes, until leaves are tender. Spread leaves; add salt, fat-free mozzarella cheese, and optional ingredients if desired. Bake at 350 degrees for 10 to 15 minutes, until cheese is totally melted.

Servings: 4
Fat: 0 g
Carbs: 16 g

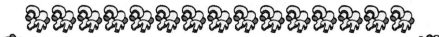

Stuffed Portabella Mushroom Caps

Ingredients

4 large portabella mushrooms
16 oz. fat-free ricotta cheese or fat-free feta cheese
12 oz. jar salsa *or* 8 cherry tomatoes *or* 1/2 pint roasted peppers
(not packed in oil)
1/3 cup fat-free mozzarella cheese
1/3 cup crabmeat or shredded chicken breast (optional)

Directions

Preheat oven at 375 degrees for 10 minutes. Spay mushrooms
on both sides with butter-flavored cooking spray and place on
baking sheet. Lower oven temperature to 350 degrees; bake for
10 minutes, top down. Turn mushrooms over and bake another
10 minutes. Remove from oven and spread cheese of your choice.
Add salsa, cherry tomatoes, or peppers, and crabmeat or chicken.
Sprinkle each mushroom with fat-free mozzarella cheese. Place
back in oven until the cheese is melted, then enjoy!

Servings: 4
Fat: 0 g
Carbs: 2 g

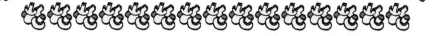

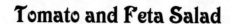

Tomato and Feta Salad

Ingredients

4 large tomatoes
6 oz. fat-free feta cheese
2 scallions
1/3 cup balsamic vinegar
Salt/pepper/oregano to taste

Directions

Slice tomatoes, chop scallions, and mix all ingredients together well in a bowl. Drizzle generously with balsamic vinegar. Feel free to substitute fat-free mozzarella for the feta!

Servings: 4
Fat: 0 g
Carbs: 5 g

Banana Cream Pie

Ingredients

16 oz. fat-free cream cheese
1/4 cup egg substitute
2/3 cup sugar-free white chocolate syrup (or sugar-free vanilla syrup)
6 oz. fat-free Greek yogurt
2 large, ripe bananas

Directions

Put all ingredients in a blender and blend until smooth. Use nonstick spray to coat a pie pan. Pour mixture into pan. Bake at 325 degrees for 1 hour, until sides separate from pan. Do not brown or overcook. Let stand for one hour to cool. Refrigerate for 2 hours before serving.

For presentation, top with fat-free whipped cream and sprinkle with chocolate shavings or decorate with fat-free/sugar-free chocolate sauce. Cinnamon is also good.

Alternately, you can make this cupcake style in 12 cupcake foils. If doing that, bake for 35 minutes and count 15 carbs per cupcake.

For peaches and cream pie, try using four peaches instead of bananas!

Servings: 8
Serving Size: 1 slice
Fat: 0 g
Carbs: 20 g

Dessert Crepe

Ingredients

4 prepackaged crepes
16 oz. fat-free ricotta cheese or fat-free Greek yogurt
1 pint fresh blueberries (feel free to use other fruits)
1/4 cup sugar-free vanilla syrup
Fat-free whipped cream

Directions

Combine ricotta cheese or yogurt in blender with fruit and sugar-free syrup. Divide between 4 crepes. Place in crepe and fold. Microwave for 20 seconds. Serve with fat-free whipped cream.

Servings: 4
Serving Size: 1 crepe
Fat per serving: 1 g
Carbs per serving: 20 g

Breakfast, Lunch, or Dinner Omelets

Ingredients

6 oz. egg whites or egg substitute
Salt/pepper to taste
1/4 cup of vegetables and cheese and/or meat
Vegetables: onions, peppers, tomatoes, mushrooms, spinach, broccoli, and/or asparagus
Cheese: fat-free feta, fat-free American, fat-free cheddar, fat-free mozzarella
Meat: Chopped Canadian bacon or bacon bits. (Need to add these to the fat count.)

Directions

If using meat or vegetables, heat small skillet on medium heat. Cover pan with cooking spray, then add your meat/vegetables and a pinch of salt and sauté about 5 minutes. Remove from pan and cover to keep meat/vegetables warm.

With the skillet still hot, spray again to coat, and add egg substitute to cover the bottom of the pan. Add salt and pepper to taste. Cook until set, about 2 minutes. Using a rubber scraper, lift the eggs up and let the runny, uncooked egg flow underneath.

Spoon your vegetables/meats/cheese onto half of the omelet, fold over, and serve on a plate.

Servings: 1
Fat: 0 g
Carbs: 5 g

Remember to count fat if adding bacon bits!

Frittata

Ingredients

12 oz. egg whites or egg substitute
1 cup fat-free cheddar cheese
1/2 tsp. black pepper
1/4 tsp. salt
Butter-flavored cooking spray
1/2 cup chopped broccoli
1/2 cup chopped and onions
1 tbsp. chopped parsley leaves

Directions

Preheat oven on broil setting. In a medium bowl, blend together egg whites/egg substitute, salt, pepper, and nonfat cheddar cheese. Add butter-flavored cooking spray onto a skillet and set on medium to high heat. Sauté broccoli and onions for 2 to 3 minutes. Pour egg mixture into the skillet, and stir with a rubber spatula. Cook for 4 to 5 minutes until the egg mixture has set on the bottom and begins to set on top. Sprinkle with parsley.

Place pan into the broiler for 3 to 4 minutes, until lightly browned and fluffy. Remove from pan and cut into 6 servings. Enjoy!

Servings: 6
Fat: 0 g
Carbs: 5 g

Cauliflower Mash

Ingredients

1 head cauliflower
6 oz. fat-free sour cream
3 tbsp. fat-free creamer
1 tsp. Butter Buds or 2 tbsp. aged balsamic vinegar
Salt/pepper to taste

Directions

Boil cauliflower in water for 10 minutes. Remove from pot, put in blender, and add the above ingredients except Butter Buds or balsamic vinegar. Blend until smooth.

Serve hot, topped with either sprinkled Butter Buds or balsamic vinegar.

Servings: 4
Fat: 0 g
Carbs: 2 g

Eggplant Marinara

Ingredients

1 eggplant
24 oz. fat-free marinara sauce
1/4 cup fat-free mozzarella cheese (optional)

Directions

Simmer eggplant in marinara sauce for 30 minutes in a sauce pot. Serve hot, at room temperature, or cold, as preferred. Feel free to melt fat-free mozzarella cheese on top to make it Parmesan style.

Great as an entrée, side dish, or topping!

Servings: 6
Fat: 0 g
Carbs: 10 g

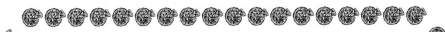

Whole-Wheat Pizza

Ingredients

1 store-bought whole-wheat pizza crust (thin crust whenever possible)
4 medium ripe red tomatoes (or 1 cup nonfat marinara sauce)
2 cups nonfat ricotta cheese
1 cup nonfat mozzarella cheese (optional)
Salt/pepper to taste
Basil, oregano, garlic, and/or parsley to taste

Directions

Preheat oven to 400 degrees. Press dough onto a nonstick pizza pan sprayed with nonstick cooking spray until the bottom is covered evenly. Spread nonfat ricotta cheese evenly onto the dough. Arrange tomato slices onto pie evenly (or spread marinara sauce).

Bake in oven for however many minutes pizza crust packaging recommends. Remove and sprinkle nonfat mozzarella cheese on top, then place back in the oven for additional 3 to 5 minutes (or until the cheese is completely melted). Remove from oven; add spices to taste.

Servings: 8
Fat: 4 g
Carbs: 30 g

Feel free to add different vegetables or even turkey pepperoni; just count any added fat.

Roasted Pineapple and Pepper Salsa

Ingredients

1/2 pineapple
1 mango, seeded
2 tbsp. lime juice
1 tbsp. chopped cilantro leaves
2 tbsp. honey
1/2 jalapeno pepper, seeded
1/2 red onion
1/2 red bell pepper, seeded
Salt to taste

Directions

Core and peel pineapple half and cut into 1/4 in. slices. Cut mango into 1/4 in. slices as well. Mince jalapeno; dice bell pepper and onion.

Spray skillet with nonstick cooking spray. Heat skillet on high. Place pineapples and mangos in skillet, sauté for 45 seconds, and remove. Let cool.

In a mixing bowl, combine honey, lime juice, and cilantro and season with salt to taste. Add the pineapple and mango. Mix well. Let sit for one hour and serve.

Great to serve with shrimp cocktail or as a topping for your entree!

Servings: approximately 40
Serving Size: 1 tbsp.
Fat: 0 g
Carbs: 5 g

Shrimp Cocktail

Ingredients

1 lemon
2 dried bay leaves
1 tbsp. mustard seed
36 large raw shrimp, peeled and deveined

Directions

Place a deep pot halfway filled with water over high heat. Squeeze the juice from the lemon into the water. Add bay leaves and mustard seed.

Once water is boiling, add shrimp, and boil for approximately 5 minutes. The shrimp should turn pink, and the tails will curl. Drain and run under cold water.

Refrigerate until ready to serve.

Servings: 6
Serving Size: 6 shrimps
Fat: 1 g
Carbs: 0 g

Great to dip in cocktail sauce or the Roasted Pineapple and Pepper Salsa from the previous page.

Spanakotyropita (Greek Spinach Pie)

Ingredients

40 oz. frozen spinach (defrosted)
1/2 package phyllo dough
2 cups fat-free feta cheese
1 large onion, chopped
3/4 cup egg whites or egg substitute
Salt/pepper to taste
Optional: 1 cup chopped mushrooms or chopped cooked chicken breast

Directions

Preheat oven to 350 degrees. In a bowl, combine spinach, feta cheese, chopped onion, and egg whites/egg substitute. If adding mushrooms or chicken, add them now too. Season with salt and pepper, and mix well.

Spray a baking pan (not smaller than 9 × 13 in.) with butter-flavored nonstick oil a baking pan. Place 4 sheets of phyllo to cover bottom. Spread half of the mixture in the bowl onto the phyllo dough evenly. Add 3 more sheets of phyllo dough on top. Spray with butter-flavored nonstick cooking spray. Add the rest of mixture evenly and place 4 layers of phyllo dough on top. Spray again with butter-flavored nonstick spray. Cover with aluminum foil.

Place pan in oven and cook covered for 30 minutes. Remove foil. Place back in oven for an additional 10 to 15 minutes until the dough on top starts to brown. Remove. Let sit for 10 minutes, then serve!

Servings: 12
Fat: 2 g
Carbs: 20 g

Remember to count fat/carbs if adding chicken or mushrooms!

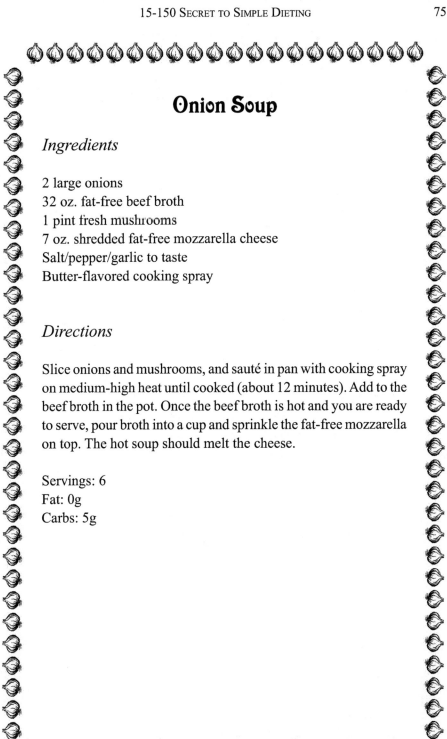

Onion Soup

Ingredients

2 large onions
32 oz. fat-free beef broth
1 pint fresh mushrooms
7 oz. shredded fat-free mozzarella cheese
Salt/pepper/garlic to taste
Butter-flavored cooking spray

Directions

Slice onions and mushrooms, and sauté in pan with cooking spray on medium-high heat until cooked (about 12 minutes). Add to the beef broth in the pot. Once the beef broth is hot and you are ready to serve, pour broth into a cup and sprinkle the fat-free mozzarella on top. The hot soup should melt the cheese.

Servings: 6
Fat: 0g
Carbs: 5g

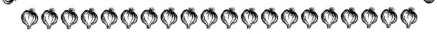

Crustless Pumpkin Pie

Ingredients

15 oz. canned pumpkin
1/2 cup egg whites or egg substitute
3/4 cup sugar substitute
2 tbsp. ground cinnamon
2 tbsp. fat-free whipped cream

Directions

Preheat oven to 350 degrees for 10 minutes. Place all ingredients except whipped cream in a bowl and mix well with a spoon. Spray baking pan with spray oil, and place mixture in pan. Bake for approximately 25 minutes. Once cooled, let sit in refrigerator for two hours. Top and serve with fat-free whipped cream and a little more sprinkled cinnamon.

Servings: 8
Fat: 1 g
Carbs: 8 g

Refried Bean Dip

Ingredients

16 oz. fat-free refried beans
16 oz. salsa, your choice: mild, medium, or hot
16 oz. fat-free sour cream or fat free cream cheese
7 oz. fat-free shredded cheddar cheese
4 scallions
8 multigrain chips (optional)

Directions

Layer refried beans, salsa, and sour cream (cream cheese), about
3/4 in. per layer, in a flat-bottomed dish. Depending on the size
of your dish, you may need to make multiple layers of each. Top
with chopped scallions and cheddar cheese.

Serve at room temperature or bake in oven at 350 degrees for 15
minutes, until cheese is well melted. Serve with slices of peppers,
celery, or green beans.

Servings: 6 to 8
Fat: 0 g
Carbs: 16 g

If you choose to dip chips, look for whole-wheat or multi-grain
chips, and count fat and carbs.

Tzatziki Sauce

Ingredients

4 medium cucumbers
1 cup fat-free Greek yogurt
1 tsp. fresh lemon juice or white wine vinegar
1/2 tsp. salt
1 tsp. dill or oregano
2 tbsp. minced garlic

Directions

Peel cucumber and chop into small pieces. Add into a bowl with the rest of the ingredients and mix well. Let chill in the refrigerator for two hours, and it's ready to serve!

Great for sandwiches and toppings on your fish, chicken, or pork!

Servings: 6
Fat: 0 g
Carbs: 2 g

Yogurt Smoothie

Ingredients

6 oz. fat-free Greek yogurt
1/4 cup sugar-free syrup, your choice of flavor
1 cup ice
Fruit (optional, see below)
Fat-free whipped cream (optional)

Directions

Blend fat-free Greek yogurt, ice, sugar-free syrup, and optionally, the fruit of your choice thoroughly. If you choose to use fruit, you must count the carbs! It's not an exact science; just use 20 carbs for the size of an apple. If you'd like, top it off with some whipped cream.

Here are some flavor combinations I enjoy: blueberries with vanilla syrup, bananas with chocolate syrup, strawberries with vanilla syrup, strawberries and banana with vanilla or chocolate syrup, and mango with vanilla syrup. Experiment and find something you love!

Servings: 1
Fat: 0 g
Carbs: 7 g base; add 3 g for whipped cream; see appendix for fruit carbohydrate values

Mini Feta and Scallion Quiches

Ingredients

1 cup chopped scallions
6 oz. egg whites or egg substitute
1/2 cup nonfat creamer
1/2 teaspoon salt
1/4 teaspoon pepper
1 cup crumbled nonfat feta cheese
Butter-flavored cooking spray

Directions

Preheat oven to 300 degrees. Sauté scallions for 10 minutes over medium heat in a skillet coated with nonstick cooking spray, then let cool. Mix egg substitute, nonfat creamer, salt, pepper, and nonfat feta cheese and scallions. Coat a mini muffin pan with butter-flavored nonstick cooking spray. Divide mixture into a mini muffin pan with a spoon. Do not fill to the top.

Bake until set, about 15 minutes. Serve warm. You can refrigerate or freeze to save for later.

Servings: 24
Fat: 0 g
Carbs: 2 g

These quiches are wonderfully versatile. You can add any vegetable, nonfat cheese, and even bacon bits or Canadian bacon. Vary the ingredients to suit your taste; just make sure to get the right fat and carb count.

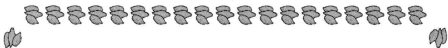

Yams

Ingredients

2 large yams
Butter-flavored cooking spray

Directions

Preheat oven to 350 degrees. Cut ends off yams and discard. Cut remaining yam centers into 1/2 in. slices. Spray both sides of each slice with butter-flavored cooking spray. Place yams on cookie sheet. Bake each side for approximately 10 to 15 minutes.

Ready to serve immediately.

Servings: approximately 8
Serving size: 1 slice
Fat: 0 g
Carbs: 15 g

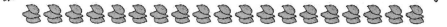

Peach Turnovers

Ingredients

1 package phyllo dough
2 fresh peaches
1/2 cup sugar-free vanilla syrup
2 tsp. cinnamon

Directions

Spray skillet with nonfat cooking spray and heat on stovetop on low-medium heat. Peel skin off peaches, and cut them into slices. Pour syrup into skillet. Place peaches in skillet and cook for approximately 10 to 15 minutes, until fruit is soft.

Preheat toaster oven to 350 degrees. Cut phyllo dough into smaller sheets of approximately 5 in. by 6 in. Put three sheets down. Add cooked fruit. Put three more sheets on top. Lightly spray top with cooking spray. Sprinkle one teaspoon of cinnamon on each serving. Bake pastries in toaster oven for 10 minutes or until phyllo becomes crisp and brown.

Serve warm and enjoy!

If you would prefer apple turnovers, substitute two apples for two peaches; just make sure to core and peel the apples.

Servings: 2
Fat: 1 g
Carbs: 35 g

APPENDIX A
BOBBIE'S SHOPPING LIST

Any project can be completed easier and faster with the right tools. In our case, foods are our tools. Below is a list of foods that have been very helpful to me in my weight-loss journey. These are good, versatile, low-fat, low-carb foods (or at least ingredients) that are each part of my day-to-day diet in their own way.

Like almost every other part of this diet, the shopping list is customizable to your taste and lifestyle. Feel free to add your own low-fat, low-carb foods to this list. If you make these foods staples of your diet, they're really going to help you lose weight.

Essentials

- Assorted fat-free cheeses
- Egg whites or egg substitutes
- Mustards of all varieties—yellow, brown, honey, and Dijon
- Jars of pickles and roasted peppers (not in oil)
- Canned tuna fish in water
- Fat-free mayo
- Fat-free tomato sauce
- Fat-free sour cream
- Veggie and salad mixes
- Balsamic vinegar
- Fresh turkey breast
- Fat-free maple ham
- Grilled chicken breast
- Shrimp cocktail
- Crabmeat
- Fresh fish of all types

- Lox, fat-free cream cheese, and chives
- Sugar-free flavored syrups
- Lots of spices, such as garlic, oregano, and parsley
- Salsa
- Sugar-free, low carb drinks
- Fat-free whipped cream
- Sugar-free gelatin
- Butter substitutes
- Fat-free creamer
- Artificial sweeteners
- Fat Free Spay Oils—I prefer the "butter" flavored.

Most of these essentials have no fat or carb content at all!

Other Great Tools

- Fat-free Greek yogurt
- Fat-free, sugar-free pudding
- Low-carb, low-fat muffins and breads
- Assorted low fat, low carb dressings and marinades for cooking.
- Fat-free refried beans
- Low-carb, low-fat soups
- Low-carb, low-fat ice cream treats
- Pumpkin, apple butter (no sugar added), and apple butter BBQ sauce.
- Natural jellies
- Phyllo dough
- Fruits
- Yams
- Canned pumpkin
- Low-carb, low-fat cookies
- Crepes
- Whole-grain pretzels
- Wasabi peas
- Popcorn (unbuttered) and fat free carmel popcorn
- Dark chocolate dessert shells

APPENDIX B
FAT AND CARB VALUES

This appendix has been developed by and large from the USDA values, supplemented where necessary or relevant by fat and carb values directly from brand-name products' nutritional labels. Although this is a rather lengthy list and thus will address many of the things you eat over the course of the day, that doesn't get you off the hook from reading labels! This is only a general guide—good as a stand-in if you don't have access to specific information for what you're eating. Different manufacturers often have different amounts of fat and carbs in the same products. Values for restaurant foods and many prepared foods can be looked up online; just plug "(name of food) nutrition data" into a search engine or go to the restaurant website and you'll find them, no problem. You have many resources easily available to you, so use them!

In this appendix, when serving sizes are listed in ounces, assume that they are ounces of weight when dealing with solids and fluid ounces when dealing with liquids or powders.

All meat and fish products are for cooked foods, where relevant, unless otherwise noted. The values for cooked meats and fish are generally for when they are dry cooked, steamed, or broiled, unless otherwise noted. As a matter of principle, fried foods should be avoided; hence, very few fried foods are listed in this appendix, as they are almost universally too fatty.

Baking Products

Item	Portion Size	Carbs (g)	Fat (g)
All-purpose white flour	1 cup	95	1
Baking chocolate (unsweetened)	1 oz.	8	15
Baking powder	1 tsp.	1	0

Baking soda	1 tsp.	0	0
Chocolate chips (semisweet)	1 oz.	18	8
Cinnamon	1 tbsp.	6	0
Cocoa powder (unsweetened)	1 oz.	16	4
Coconut milk	1 cup	6	48
Coconut (dried, unsweetened)	1 oz.	7	18
Gelatin	1 tbsp.	0	0
Margarine	1 tsp.	0	4
Molasses	1 tbsp.	15	0
Sugar (brown)	1 tsp.	4	0
Sugar (white)	1 tsp.	4	0

Beverages

Item	Portion Size	Carbs (g)	Fat (g)
Acai juice	1 cup	23	0
Apple juice	1 cup	9	0
Cranberry juice (unsweetened)	1 cup	31	0
Cranberry juice cocktail	1 cup	34	0
Grapefruit juice	1 cup	22	0
Grape juice	1 cup	37	0
Lemon juice	1 oz.	3	0
Lime juice	1 oz.	3	0
Orange juice	1 cup	25	1
Pomegranate juice	1 cup	33	1
Tomato juice	1 cup	10	0
V-8	1 cup	10	0
Chocolate milk	1 cup	26	8
Hot cocoa	1 cup	27	6
Coffee (black, unsweetened)	1 cup	0	0
Tea (unsweetened)	1 cup	0	0
VitaminWater	1 cup	13	0
Gatorade	1 cup	14	0
Coca-Cola	1 cup	27	0
Diet Coke	1 cup	0	0
Pepsi	1 cup	27	0
Diet Pepsi	1 cup	0	0

Beer	12 oz.	13	0
Light beer	12 oz.	7	0
Bourbon	1 oz.	0	0
Brandy	1 oz.	0	0
Gin	1 oz.	0	0
Red wine	5 oz.	4	0
White wine	5 oz.	4	0
White wine (Riesling)	5 oz.	6	0
Rum	1 oz.	0	0
Scotch	1 oz.	0	0
Tequila	1 oz.	0	0
Triple sec	1 oz.	11	0
Vodka	1 oz.	0	0
Whiskey	1 oz.	0	0

Breads/Rolls/Crackers

Item	Portion Size	Carbs (g)	Fat (g)
Bagel (plain, onion, sesame, or poppy)	1 bagel	29	1
Cinnamon raisin bagel	1 bagel	31	1
Biscuit	1 biscuit	17	6
Blueberry muffin	1 small muffin	33	13
Bran muffin	1 muffin	19	3
Breadsticks	1 breadstick	8	0
Corn muffin	1 muffin	29	4
Cornbread	1 piece	28	5
Graham crackers	4 crackers	11	1
Ritz crackers	5 crackers	10	4
Rye wafer crackers	5 crackers	45	0
Saltine crackers	5 crackers	10	1
Water crackers	5 crackers	15	1
Croissant	1 croissant	26	12
English muffin	1 muffin	27	1
Hard white roll	1 roll	30	2
Italian bread	1 slice	15	1
Pita	1 pita	33	1
Popover	1 piece	9	4

Item	Portion Size	Total Carbs (g)	Fat (g)
Pumpernickel bread	1 slice	12	1
Raisin bread	1 slice	17	1
Rye bread	1 slice	15	1
Soft hoagie roll	1 roll	35	6
Sourdough bread	1 slice	18	1
Corn tortilla	1 tortilla	11	1
Flour tortilla	1 tortilla	24	4
Wheat bread	1 slice	12	1
White bread	1 slice	13	1
Whole grain bread	1 slice	11	1
French toast (frozen)	1 slice	19	4
French toast (homemade)	1 slice	16	7
Pancakes (frozen)	1 pancake	30	4
Pancakes (homemade)	1 pancake	22	7
Waffles (frozen)	1 waffle	15	3
Waffles (homemade)	1 waffle	25	11

Cereals and Oatmeal

Item	Portion Size	Total Carbs (g)	Fat (g)
Cream of rice cereal (cooked)	1 cup	28	0
Cream of wheat cereal (cooked)	1 cup	32	1
Oatmeal (cooked)	1 cup	56	5
Apple Jacks	1 cup	30	0
Cheerios	1 cup	21	2
Multi-Grain Cheerios	1 cup	25	1
Chex	1 cup	26	1
Cocoa Puffs	1 cup	26	2
Corn flakes	1 cup	24	1
Froot Loops	1 cup	26	1
Frosted flakes	0.75 cup	27	0
Grape nuts	0.5 cup	48	1
Raisin bran	0.5 cup	23	1
Rice Krispies	1 cup	24	0
Wheaties	1 cup	24	1

Dairy, Including Cheese

Item	Portion Size	Carbs (g)	Fat (g)
Butter	1 tbsp.	0	11
Butter (whipped)	1 tbsp.	0	8
Buttermilk (1 percent)	1 cup	12	2
Half and half	1 oz.	1	3
Heavy whipping cream	1 tbsp.	0	11
Milk (whole)	1 cup	13	8
Milk (2 percent)	1 cup	14	5
Milk (1 percent)	1 cup	14	3
Milk (skim)	1 cup	12	0
Sour cream	1 oz.	1	6
Yogurt (low-fat, plain)	1 cup	17	4
Yogurt (fat-free/skim, plain)	1 cup	19	0
Yogurt (whole milk, plain)	1 cup	11	8
American cheese	1 oz.	3	4
Blue cheese	1 oz.	1	8
Cheddar (shredded)	1 oz.	0	9
Cream cheese	1 tbsp.	1	5
Cottage cheese (1 percent)	0.5 cup	3	1
Feta (crumbled)	1 oz.	1	6
Fontina (shredded)	1 oz.	9	9
Goat cheese (soft)	1 oz.	0	6
Goat cheese (hard)	1 oz.	1	10
Mascarpone	1 oz.	1	13
Manchego	1 oz.	0	10
Monterey cheese	1 oz.	0	8
Mozzarella (whole milk)	1 oz.	1	6
Mozzarella (skim milk)	1 oz.	1	4
Mozzarella (fat-free)	1 oz.	1	0
Muenster	1 oz.	0	8
Parmesan cheese (grated)	1 oz.	1	8
Provolone	1 oz.	1	7
Ricotta (whole milk)	1 oz.	1	4
Romano	1 oz.	1	8
Swiss cheese	1 oz.	2	8
Velveeta	1 oz.	3	6

Desserts and Pastries

Item	Portion Size	Carbs (g)	Fat (g)
Angel food cake	1 slice (3 oz.)	49	0
Chocolate layer cake	1 slice (3 oz.)	42	13
Coffee cake	1 cake (2 oz.)	27	13
Pound cake	1 slice (1 oz.)	15	6
Brownie	2 oz.	36	9
Dark chocolate	1 oz.	17	9
Milk chocolate	1 oz.	17	8
Chocolate chip cookie	1 cookie	8	3
Gingersnaps	1 cookie	5	1
Oatmeal cookie	1 cookie	17	5
Peanut butter cookie	1 cookie	9	4
Sugar cookie	1 cookie	10	3
Plain donut	1 doughnut	19	11
Glazed donut	1 doughnut	27	14
Jelly doughnut	1 doughnut	25	12
Chocolate ice cream	0.5 cup	18	7
Strawberry ice cream	0.5 cup	16	5
Vanilla ice cream	0.5 cup	16	7
Apple pie	1/8 of 9" pie	42	14
Cherry pie	1/8 of 9" pie	50	14
Lemon meringue pie	1/8 of 9" pie	53	10
Pecan pie	1/8 of 9" pie	79	22
Pumpkin pie	1/8 of 9" pie	46	13
Jell-O	21 g.	19	0

Eggs

Item	Portion Size	Carbs (g)	Fat (g)
Egg white	1 egg white	0	0
Egg yolk	1 egg yolk	1	5
Egg (whole, fresh)	1 egg	1	5
Egg Beaters	0.25 cup	1	0

Fruit and Fruit Products

Item	Portion Size	Carbs (g)	Fat (g)
Apple	1 fruit	25	0
Applesauce (sweetened)	0.5 cup	26	0
Applesauce (unsweetened)	0.5 cup	14	0
Apricots (dried)	0.25 cup	20	0
Apricots (fresh)	1 fruit	4	0
Avocado	1 fruit	17	29
Banana	1 fruit	27	0
Blackberries	1 cup	15	1
Blueberries	1 cup	21	0
Cantaloupe (cubed)	1 cup	14	0
Cherries (sweet)	1 cup, with pits	22	0
Cherries (sour)	1 cup, with pits	13	0
Cranberries (dried, sweetened)	1 cup	33	1
Cranberries (fresh)	1 cup	12	0
Currants (dried)	0.25 cup	27	0
Dates	0.25 cup	27	1
Figs (fresh)	1 large fruit	12	0
Figs (dried)	0.25 cup	24	0
Grapes	1 cup	27	0
Honeydew	1 cup	16	0
Kiwi	1 fruit	13	0
Mango (sliced)	1 cup	28	0
Nectarine	1 fruit	15	0
Orange	1 fruit	18	0
Papaya	1 cup	14	0
Peach	1 fruit	17	0
Pear	1 fruit	23	0
Pineapple (chunks)	1 cup	22	0
Plum	1 fruit	8	0
Pomegranate	0.5 cup arils	16	1
Prunes (pitted)	0.25 cup	27	0
Raspberries	1 cup	15	1
Raisins	0.25 cup	33	1
Strawberries	1 cup	12	0
Tangerine	1 fruit	12	0
Watermelon	1 cup	12	0

Grains

Item	Portion Size	Carbs (g)	Fat (g)
Bulgur (cooked)	0.5 cup	17	0
Cornmeal	1 oz.	22	1
Couscous (cooked)	0.5 cup	18	0
Hominy (canned)	0.5 cup	12	0.5
Kasha (cooked)	0.5 cup	17	1
Millet (cooked)	0.5 cup	21	1
Oat bran (cooked)	0.5 cup	13	1
Barley (pearled, cooked)	0.5 cup	22	0.5
Quinoa (cooked)	0.5 cup	20	2
Brown rice (cooked)	0.5 cup	23	1
White rice (cooked)	0.5 cup	19	0
Wild rice (cooked)	0.5 cup	18	0.5
Wheat germ (crude)	0.25 cup	15	3

Lunch Meat

Item	Portion Size	Carbs (g)	Fat (g)
Beef bologna	3 oz.	1	24
Pork bologna	3 oz.	0	18
Turkey bologna	3 oz.	1	12
Beef pastrami	3 oz.	0	6
Deli ham	3 oz.	3	8
Deli roast beef	6 oz.	0	5
Prosciutto	6 oz.	0	13
Beef salami	3 oz.	1	18
Pork salami	3 oz.	1	30
Turkey breast	3 oz.	0	6
Turkey roll	3 oz.	1	6

Beef & Veal

Item	Portion Size	Carbs (g)	Fat (g)
Beef brisket	6 oz.	0	42
Beef chuck	6 oz.	0	18
Beef eye round	6 oz.	0	16

Beef jerky	1 oz.	3	7
Beef short ribs	6 oz.	0	72
Beef tenderloin	6 oz.	0	18
Ground beef chuck (browned)	6 oz.	0	30
Ground beef round (browned)	6 oz.	0	26
Calf liver	6 oz.	11	10
Corned beef brisket	6 oz.	0	32
Cube steak	6 oz.	0	11
Filet mignon	6 oz.	0	15
Beef hot dog	1 hot dog (no bun)	2	13
Ground veal	6 oz.	0	12
Prime rib	6 oz.	0	34
Rib eye	6 oz.	0	15
Shell steak	6 oz.	0	34
Sirloin steak	6 oz.	0	26
Skirt steak	6 oz.	0	20
Top loin	6 oz.	0	28
Top sirloin	6 oz.	0	24
Veal arm shoulder	6 oz.	0	14
Veal breast	6 oz.	0	28
Veal cutlet	6 oz.	0	20
Veal loin	6 oz.	0	20
Veal rib chop	6 oz.	0	24
Veal round steak	6 oz.	0	7
Veal shank	6 oz.	0	10
Veal (cubed for stew)	6 oz.	0	8

Lamb

Item	*Portion Size*	*Carbs (g)*	*Fat (g)*
Ground lamb	6 oz.	0	34
Lamb rib chops	6 oz.	0	46
Lamb shoulder	6 oz.	0	38
Lamb stew meat	6 oz.	0	12
Leg of lamb (bone-in)	6 oz.	0	20
Rack of lamb	6 oz.	0	20

Pork

Item	Portion Size	Carbs (g)	Fat (g)
Bacon	3 pieces	0	9
Canadian bacon	3 pieces	1	6
Ground pork	6 oz.	0	36
Ham (boneless)	6 oz.	0	12
Kielbasa	1 link	2	20
Pancetta	1 oz.	0	9
Pork chop (center cut)	6 oz.	0	9
Pork hot dog	1 hot dog (no bun)	0	18
Pork loin chops	6 oz.	0	18
Pork loin roast	6 oz.	0	26
Pork loin (boneless)	6 oz.	0	8
Pork sausage	2 oz.	0	16
Pork spareribs	6 oz.	0	51
Pork tenderloin	6 oz.	0	14

Poultry

Item	Portion Size	Carbs (g)	Fat (g)
Chicken breast (skinless)	6 oz.	0	3
Chicken leg (skinless)	1 leg	0	8
Chicken liver pate	2 tbsp.	2	4
Chicken thigh	1 thigh	0	6
Chicken wing	1 wing	0	2
Ground chicken	6 oz.	0	18
Chicken hot dog	1 hot dog (no bun)	1	7
Chicken/turkey sausage	1 link	7	12
Cornish game hen (skinless)	1/2 bird	0	4
Duck breast (skinless)	6 oz.	0	4
Duck (whole)	6 oz.	0	25
Goose (whole)	6 oz.	0	36
Turkey breast cutlet	6 oz.	0	1
Turkey breast (skinless, boneless)	6 oz.	0	2
Turkey hot dog	1 hot dog (no bun)	2	8
Turkey (ground)	6 oz.	0	22
Turkey (whole)	6 oz.	0	17

Seafood

Item	Portion Size	Carbs (g)	Fat (g)
Anchovies (boneless, in oil, canned, drained)	1 oz.	0	3
Bluefish	6 oz.	0	10
Catfish	6 oz.	0	14
Clams (canned, drained)	6 oz.	8	4
Cod	6 oz.	0	2
Conch	6 oz.	2	2
Crab meat	6 oz.	0	2
Halibut	6 oz.	0	4
Lobster meat	6 oz.	1	1
Mackerel	6 oz.	0	30
Mahi mahi	6 oz.	0	2
Mussels	6 oz.	12	8
Oysters	6 oz.	8	4
Salmon steak	6 oz.	0	20
Smoked salmon (lox)	3 oz.	0	4
Scallops	6 oz.	4	2
Scrod	6 oz.	0	1
Sea bass	6 oz.	0	4
Shrimp	6 oz.	0	2
Snapper	6 oz.	0	2
Squid (fried calamari)	3 oz.	7	6
Trout	6 oz.	0	14
Tuna (whole)	6 oz.	0	10
Tuna (canned, oil-packed)	3 oz.	0	7
Tuna (canned, water-packed)	3 oz.	0	1

Oils/Salad Dressings

Item	Portion Size	Carbs (g)	Fat (g)
Corn oil	1 tsp.	0	5
Peanut oil	1 tsp.	0	5
Olive oil	1 tsp.	0	5
Sesame oil	1 tsp.	0	5
Blue cheese dressing	2 tbsp.	2	16

Caesar dressing	2 tbsp.	1	17
Italian dressing	2 tbsp.	4	8
Ranch dressing	2 tbsp.	2	16
Thousand Island dressing	2 tbsp.	5	11
French dressing	2 tbsp.	6	14
Russian dressing	2 tbsp.	10	8
Vinaigrette dressing	2 tbsp.	4	8

Nuts/Seeds (raw unless otherwise noted)

Item	Portion Size	Carbs (g)	Fat (g)
Almond butter	2 tbsp.	6	19
Almonds	1 oz. (23 kernels)	6	14
Chestnuts (roasted)	1 oz. (3 kernels)	15	1
Hazelnuts	10 nuts	2	9
Macadamia nuts	5 kernels	2	11
Peanut butter	2 tbsp.	7	16
Peanuts	14 nuts	3.4	8.9
Pecans	0.5 oz. (10 halves)	2	10
Pine nuts	0.5 oz. (80 kernels)	2	10
Pistachios	0.5 oz. (25 kernels)	4	7
Pumpkin seeds (hulled)	0.5 oz. (70 seeds)	3	7
Soy nuts	1 oz.	9	6
Sunflower seeds	1 oz.	6	14
Walnuts (halved)	0.5 oz. (7 halves)	2	9

Pasta

Item	Portion Size	Carbs (g)	Fat (g)
Egg noodles (cooked)	0.5 cup	20	1.5
Spinach pasta (cooked)	0.5 cup	14	1
Whole wheat pasta (cooked)	0.5 cup	19	1
Pasta (fresh, cooked)	0.5 cup	20	0.5

Sauces/Gravies/Condiments

Item	Portion Size	Carbs (g)	Fat (g)
Alfredo sauce	0.25 cup	5	11
Au jus	0.25 cup	2	0
Barbeque sauce	2 tbsp.	13	0

Cranberry sauce (canned)	1 slice (0.5 in.)	22	0
Fish sauce	1 tsp.	1	0
Beef gravy	0.5 cup	6	2.5
Chicken gravy	0.5 cup	7	7
Turkey gravy	0.5 cup	6	2.5
Cocktail sauce	0.5 cup	12	0
Hollandaise sauce	0.5 cup	5	1
Honey	1 tbsp.	17	0
Horseradish (prepared)	1 tbsp.	2	0
Jam/preserves	1 tbsp.	14	0
Jelly	1 tbsp.	15	0
Ketchup	1 tbsp.	4	0
Mayonnaise	1 tsp.	0	4
Dijon mustard	1 tsp.	2	1
Honey mustard	1 tsp.	2	0
Yellow mustard	1 oz.	1	1
Pickle relish	1 tbsp.	5	0
Salsa	1 tbsp.	1	0
Sauerkraut	0.5 cup	4	0
Soy sauce	1 tbsp.	1	0
Spaghetti/marinara sauce	0.5 cup	18	3.5
Sweet & sour sauce	0.25 cup	10	0
Tartar sauce	1 oz.	1	18
Teriyaki sauce	1 tbsp.	3	0
Tomato sauce	0.25 cup	5	0
Balsamic vinegar	1 tbsp.	3	0
Cider vinegar	1 tbsp.	0	0
Distilled vinegar	1 tbsp.	0	0
Red wine vinegar	1 tbsp.	0	0
Rice vinegar (seasoned)	1 tbsp.	1	0
Sherry vinegar	1 tbsp.	4	0
Maple syrup	1 tbsp.	13	0
Pancake syrup	1 tbsp.	14	0
Vodka sauce	0.25 cup	4	7
Worcestershire sauce	1 tbsp.	3	0

Soups (prepared, not condensed)

Item	Portion Size	Carbs (g)	Fat (g)
Beef broth	1 cup	1	0
Chicken broth	1 cup	1	1
Black bean soup	1 cup	19	2
Borscht	1 cup	9	1.5
Chicken noodle soup	1 cup	7	2
Clam chowder	1 cup	12	2
Cream of mushroom soup	1 cup	7	8
Cream of potato soup	1 cup	11	2
Egg drop soup	1 cup	10	1
Gazpacho	1 cup	4	0
Gumbo	1 cup	8	1
Lentil soup (with ham)	1 cup	20	3
Minestrone	1 cup	11	3
Miso	1 cup	73	17
Onion soup	1 cup	8	2
Split-pea soup (with ham)	1 cup	28	4
Tomato bisque	1 cup	24	3
Tomato soup	1 cup	16	1
Vegetable soup	1 cup	19	3.7
Wonton soup	1 cup	12	1

Spices/Herbs

Item	Portion Size	Carbs (g)	Fat (g)
Capers	1 tbsp.	0	0
Chili powder	1 tbsp.	4	1
Cumin	1 tbsp.	3	1
Dill pickle	1 pickle.	3	0
Garlic (fresh)	3 cloves	3	0
Ginger root slices	5 slices	2	0
Miso paste	1 tbsp.	5	1
Black olives	10 small olives	2	3
Green olives (with/without pimento)	10 olives	2	4
Pesto	1 tbsp.	1	7

Tahini	1 tbsp.	4	7
Basil (fresh)	1 tbsp.	0	0
Chives (fresh)	1 tbsp.	0	0
Cilantro (Chinese parsley)	1 tbsp.	0	0
Dill seed	1 tbsp.	4	1
Parsley (fresh)	1 tbsp.	0	0
Sage (ground)	1 tbsp.	1	0
Rosemary (fresh)	1 tbsp.	0	0
Thyme (fresh)	1 tbsp.	1	0
Paprika (ground)	1 tbsp.	4	1
Oregano (dried)	1 tsp.	1	0

Vegetarian

Item	Portion Size	Carbs (g)	Fat (g)
Soy milk	8 oz.	15	4
Tofu (firm)	3 oz.	7	3
Tofu (silken)	3 oz.	2	2
Tofurkey	4 oz.	10	5
Veggie burger (without bun)	1 patty	10	4

Vegetables (raw unless otherwise noted)

Item	Portion Size	Carbs (g)	Fat (g)
Artichoke	1 vegetable	13	0
Artichoke heart	3 hearts	1	2
Asparagus	1 cup	5	0
Green beans	0.5 cup	5	0
Bok choy	1 cup	2	0
Broccoflower	0.5 cup	4	0
Broccoli (chopped)	1 cup	6	0
Broccoli rabe (cooked)	3 oz.	3	0
Brussels sprouts	1 cup	8	0
Cabbage	1 cup	5	0
Savoy cabbage	1 cup	4	0
Red cabbage	1 cup	7	0
Carrot	1 vegetable	7.3	0.1

Cauliflower	1 cup	5	0
Celery	0.5 cup	4	0
Collards	1 cup	2	0
Corn (yellow)	1 medium ear	17	1
Cucumber (peeled)	1 cup	3	0
Daikon	3 oz.	4	0
Eggplant (cubed)	1 cup	5	0
Endive	0.5 cup	1	0
Fennel	0.5 cup	3	0
Mixed greens	1 cup	2	0
Jicama/yambean (sliced)	1 cup	11	0
Kale	0.5 cup	4	0
Leeks	1 vegetable	13	0
Lettuce (shredded)	1 cup	1	0
Portabella mushrooms	1 mushroom	4	0
White mushrooms	1 cup	2	0
Shiitake mushrooms	4 mushrooms	11	0
Okra	1 cup	7	0
Onions (chopped)	1 cup	15	0
Peas (green)	0.5 cup	10	0.5
Chili pepper	1 vegetable	4	0
Green pepper	1 vegetable	6	0
Red pepper	1 vegetable	7	0
Jalapeno pepper	1 cup	6	1
Roasted pepper	1 oz.	1	0
Sweet potato	1 vegetable	26	0
White potato	0.5 cup	13	0
Pumpkin	1 cup	8	0
Radicchio	1 cup	2	0
Radishes	0.5 cup	2	0
Rhubarb	0.5 cup	3	0
Shallots	1 tbsp.	2	0
Spinach	1 cup	1	0
Acorn squash	1 cup	15	0
Butternut squash	1 cup	16	0
Spaghetti squash	1 cup	7	1

Summer squash	1 cup	4	0
Zucchini	1 vegetable	7	0
Swiss chard	0.5 cup	1	0
Tomatillos	0.5 cup	4	1
Plum tomatoes	1 vegetable	2	0
Cherry tomatoes	1 cup	6	0
Tomatoes (canned)	0.5 cup	5	0
Sun-dried tomatoes	0.25 cup	8	0.5
Sun-dried tomatoes (oil-packed)	0.25 cup	6	4
Turnips	0.5 cup	4	0
Water chestnuts	0.5 cup	8	0
Watercress	0.5 cup	0	0

Beans (cooked)

Item	Portion Size	Carbs (g)	Fat (g)
Baby lima beans	0.5 cup	17	0.5
Black beans	0.5 cup	21	0.5
Black-eyed peas	0.5 cup	16	0
California red kidney beans	0.5 cup	20	0
Chickpea/Garbanzo beans	0.5 cup	27	3
Great northern beans	0.5 cup	19	1
Hummus	2 tbsp.	4	2
Lentils	0.5 cup	20	1
Navy beans	0.5 cup	24	1
Pink beans	0.5 cup	24	1
Pinto beans	0.5 cup	27	1
Soybeans	0.5 cup	10	6

Snacks

Item	Portion Size	Carbs (g)	Fat (g)
Potato chips	1 oz.	8	6
Sweet potato chips	1 oz.	18	7
Pretzels (soft)	1 small pretzel	43	2
Pretzels (hard)	10 pretzels	48	2
Tortilla chips	1 oz.	18	7
Cheese puffs	0.5 oz. (16 pieces)	8	5
Doritos	1 oz.	17	8

Prepared Foods

Item	Portion Size	Carbs (g)	Fat (g)
Chicken salad	3 oz.	11	9
Egg salad	3 oz.	4	13
Tuna salad	3 oz.	8	8
Hamburger (plain)	1 burger	32	23
Cheeseburger (plain)	1 burger	35	28
Chicken nuggets (breaded, fried)	6 nuggets	16	18
Macaroni and cheese	8 oz.	26	6

Contact information:

Steven Rosenberg, PhD—*DRSMROSENBERG@aol.com*

Bobbie Freiberg—*RethinkDieting@aol.com*

Website: *www.15-150Diet.com*